11-1-73

HOW TO GET YOUR MONEY'S WORTH OUT OF PSYCHIATRY

HOW TO GET YOUR MONEY'S WORTH OUT OF PSYCHIATRY

Herbert R. Lazarus, M.D.
with assistance from
Alamo Reaves

SHERBOURNE PRESS, INC.   LOS ANGELES

Library of Congress Catalog Card Number 72-96514

ISBN 0-8202-0129-4
FIRST PRINTING

Manufactured in the United States of America
by The Maple Press Company,
York, PA

1781580

ACKNOWLEDGMENTS

I AM GRATEFUL for the invaluable assistance of the following people: Alamo Reaves who assisted with the planning and writing of the manuscript, Bettie Mulvihill for clerical assistance beyond the call of duty, Marjorie Lazarus for her patience, criticism, and support when I despaired of ever completing the job to my satisfaction, and Rose Lazarus who provided the original inspiration.

PROLOGUE

MASTERING THE ART as well as the science of psychiatry has not come easily to me. Despite excellent supervision during my formative years, I was slow to acquire the kind of expertise in the field which I so fervently sought. A psychiatrist, above all else, is a clinician —one who avoids all the pat and phoney answers to life's problems. He must be able to see things in perspective in such a way that he can clarify the real issues underlying the patient's problems and not get bogged down in all sorts of irrelevant matters. The nature of life in our society is extremely complex—so complex that many people cannot keep up with it. The psychiatrist, perhaps more than anyone else, must be able to reduce life to its simplest terms and, in the context of the doctor-patient relationship, provide the kind of feedback that will best enable the patient to master his underlying anxieties as well as understand the sources of his depression and confusion.

My observations over the past fifteen years have confirmed, over and over again, that most psychiatrists have not been able to meet this challenge. This is especially true now—when Washington and all state governments are pouring billions of dollars into the system for delivering psychiatric services. As if, somehow, spending more money to provide care for more patients magically improves the quality of that care. The gullible public pays many more billions in the quest for competent psychiatric services but is being terribly stymied in this pursuit by the shroud of secrecy and lack of honesty that hovers over the field. I wrote this book to clarify the nature of the problems and to point out, for the benefit of the public: first, what distinguishes competent from incompetent psychiatry; second, who really needs and can benefit from it; third, how to go about selecting a psychiatrist; and fourth, how to facilitate the therapy once it has begun.

In addition, I have tried to answer all the questions that are bound to arise in people's minds when they consider what is involved in the search for competent psychiatric help. Having been asked these questions so many times by so many people—both patients and nonpatients—it seemed especially appropriate to set it all down in a way that would make sense, not only for myself, but for the millions of people who are asking these very same questions. Contrary to popular opinion, quality psychiatry does not have to cost a lot; it does not require a great deal of time, and it does not involve endless dwelling on irrelevant detail. It is inexpensive, of short duration, and deals only with relevant issues. Furthermore, hospitalization can be avoided in most cases. Though we are still in the minority, psychiatrists who believe thusly are gradually changing the shape and substance of psychiatric practice in America today.

CHAPTER 1

Billion Dollar Blunderbuss

LAST WEEK A woman came into my office to make an appointment. "How much do you charge?" she asked.

"Thirty-five dollars an hour," I replied.

She paled noticeably and gasped. "Thirty-five dollars! But that's so expensive!"

"Not really," I said. "In some areas psychiatrists get as much as fifty dollars an hour."

"That's downright robbery," she replied, and walked out.

I couldn't really blame her. Good psychotherapy is so beautiful, so unique in its ability to better the human situation, that I would even suggest that when conducted properly it is priceless. The unhappy fact is that very little quality psychiatry is being practiced in this country today. Most of what is being palmed off on the public as psychotherapy isn't worth five dollars an hour, much less fifty. Gullible people go on buying anyway, falling for all the phoney packaging in a medical frame of reference and assuming on the basis of faith alone that psychiatry will wave some kind of magic wand and cure them of all their ills.

Well, this just isn't the way it is. Psychiatry as a clinical practice is doing precious little for mental illness these days. The whole damn field of mental health is in the throes of a kind of professional upheaval, an internal disorganization in which the public is victim rather than victor. Money is changing hands so rapidly that no one knows where it went or how to account for it. The following figures are only rough estimates because the bureaucracy itself doesn't know how much it is spending.

In the United States last year, *several billion dollars* were spent for psychiatric services. Of that amount, approximately 20 percent was paid for private care. Forty percent more was doled out by county, state, and federal governments for public mental health care. Twenty percent was invested by the federal government in training and research. Private and state hospitals took another 10 percent for patient care, expansion, maintenance, etc. The final portion went to various other facilities with some kind of mental health label attached. Where did all this money come from and how much was accomplished by its expenditure? More to the point, was anything accomplished?

There are no reliable statistics on how many mentally ill patients were cured or improved last year, or any year for that matter. Whether a patient's fluctuating mental and emotional state has improved or deteriorated is the decision of his therapist and, sordid as it may sound, many therapists in this country are not capable of making such a judgment. Furthermore, while some patients may improve in some ways and be recorded as such on the medical records, they may deteriorate in other ways with no notation being made. Other patients may be considered better by some psychiatrists and worse by others, depending on the criteria used.

As in so much of psychiatry, there is no formal, established standard for appraising clinical therapy and its results. Because psychiatry is not a cut and dried science, it cannot formulate any really valid statistics or methodology. Without any comprehensive guide, psychiatrists are forced into the controversial realm of their own intuitions and subjective opinions—a ridiculous situation and one that's getting the field into a heap of trouble. With only my own observation and opinion as barometers, I would estimate that less than 30 percent of all mental patients treated last year truly improved and less than 15 percent, or one half of those, will actually be free of serious illness for five or more years.

In the area of training and research, the figures are a little more exact. Four hundred and sixty-seven doctors completed psychiatric residencies last year and began the practice of psychiatry. Of course, this figure doesn't reflect the quality of their education or whether they are any good as therapists. It doesn't tell the public how many incompetent people are getting into the field because of the terrible need for somebody—anybody—to fill residency posts and to do all the menial but necessary things that psychiatric residents must do because no one else is available. It doesn't mention that there is a lack of competition for psychiatric residencies, which does not exist among the more glamorous medical specialties such as surgery. It doesn't admit that any medical school graduate, no matter how lousy he was in school, how little talent he has to offer, or how indifferent he may be to the role of headshrinker, can always knock down a residency somewhere and become a psychiatrist.

The research figure doesn't say much more. It doesn't say what kind of research was being performed, whether it was worthwhile or conclusive, or if it contributed clinically to the field. It doesn't tell whether realistic and progressive research is being encouraged or whether the majority of studies being financed are pedestrian and unproductive. It doesn't give a breakdown of all the time and money wasted annually on mediocre and meaningless projects, the oceans of empty plans and reports, the vast wasteland that exists between theoretical concept and actual clinical situation.

How about the money spent in hospitals? Was it necessary? Some of it, probably. Was it well spent? Were the maximum number of patients treated with the minimum expenditure? I doubt it; in fact, I'm convinced that hospitals are inefficient. The insurance problem alone stifles effective use and economic operation of all our hospitals and especially our psychiatric facilities. Medicare, for example, recently eliminated nursing homes from its provisions so that now, instead of a psychiatric patient being in the hospital for a couple of weeks and then in a less expensive nursing home facility for the remainder of his convalescence, he must be kept in the hospital for the full time.

What about the part spent for further development of facilities? Since the advent of community psychiatry during the sixties, local, state, and federal officials have earmarked fantastic sums for public mental health facilities. Long-range individual analysis is out and crisis intervention is the new byword. Get more buildings up, hire more personnel, pour more patients through the therapeutic gates! The latest dollar-digesters in this program are the suicide prevention centers. Quantities of federal monies have been spent by the National Institute of Mental Health (NIMH) to develop these centers, and yet Edwin S. Schneidman, the guy who came up with the idea, is the first to admit that no one really knows whether or not suicide can be prevented, or even if there is a way of finding out. Therefore, these centers are worth very little as suicide prevention centers. They might have been worth something in terms of crisis intervention, but since their personnel are not adequately trained, they have ended up merely as referral centers. They are just one more expensive fad in the haphazard development of psychiatry, brought into existence by overworked people at already existing psychiatric facilities to raise more money to hire more people to answer more telephones—because telephones at these places are always ringing and maybe, in some mysterious way, just having someone answer the phone might do somebody some good. Well, maybe it does and maybe it doesn't.

Every mental patient is theoretically suicidal, if there is any degree of depression involved, and I don't ever remember seeing a patient who didn't have some degree of depression. To isolate the suicidal patient from all other patients is theoretically and practically nonsense. So the public is not getting its money's worth out of suicide prevention centers, or a lot of other public mental health facilities for that matter.

What all this is leading up to, of course, is a full-blown indictment of the rampant chaos that is the field of psychiatry today, a chaos being financed by you, the taxpayer, the fee payer, the willing contributor. At a time when population and pollution, technology and revolution are crashing through our society like tidal waves and swelling the ranks of the mentally disturbed to record proportions, when drug addiction is out of control, when homosexuality and other characterological disorders are rife, when ghettos are spewing out social deviants like lava out of volcanoes, psychiatry is fluttering around the morass like a little lost sailboat, with no direction, no stability, not much idea where it has come from, and no idea where it is going. Of course, the public isn't aware of this. The poor, innocent, ignorant, unwary man on the street is just a victim—a victim of his neuroses and psychoses, a victim of psychiatry's mass extravagance, mass incompetence, and, worst of all, mass silence on the subject.

Despite all the publicity psychiatry has received in the communications media, there is still a thick shroud of secrecy surrounding the whole unfathomable field. For that matter, there isn't much communication going on among those of us hovering like some kind of mystics under the shroud. This secrecy, this failure to discuss openly among ourselves, among patients, among interested laymen, the basic tenets of psychiatry is one of the things holding back progress in the field. Two psychiatrists in a professional confrontation can't begin to discuss the relevant clinical issues in practical terms. They get all hung up on their own little theories and resentments and end up conversing in vague pseudoterms and subtle nuances instead of getting down to the nitty-gritty of what's wrong with the patient and what will make him better. There is practically no such thing as teamwork or consultation among psychiatrists. Each doctor goes his own way, and whether his patients get better or worse is his own business.

Furthermore, it's almost impossible for one therapist to observe what another therapist is doing with his patients, even on the residency level. It's unheard of; it's like the confessional; no one else is allowed in. No one can criticize, and few are really willing to learn from another doctor's methods.

What kind of scientific progress can be accomplished under these circumstances? No meaningful contribution to human progress can be made until psychiatry crawls out from under the semireligious aura that it has wrapped around itself and allows research and therapy to be conducted on a practical, observable, common-sense basis. No one is going to get his full dollar value out of psychiatry unless he fully understands that the field is in a state of utter confusion and is willing to battle the resulting turbulence to find out just what is available in the way of quality psychotherapeutic treatment.

WHAT IS PSYCHIATRY ANYWAY?

That's a good question and, believe it or not, no two psychiatrists would answer it in the same way. This is one of the biggest problems in the field. No one knows quite where it's at, what it's supposed to be doing and, most important, what its limitations are. Theoretically, psychiatry is the branch of medicine that deals with the various disturbances in the mental and emotional functioning of individuals. On the face of it, that sounds pretty clear-cut. In actual practice, however, psychiatry is a conglomeration of approaches to many kinds of human problems and disorders—emotional, social legal, political, religious, and, well, the list seems endless.

In addition, probably no two psychiatrists would approach any given problem in exactly the same way. Probably no two human problems are exactly alike. Definitely, no two patients would respond in the same way to any one psychiatrist. These things alone place psychiatry in a unique position among other branches of medicine, making it mandatory for psychiatrists to describe their capabilities and services in terms of their own area of competence. Since psychiatry hasn't even come up with a universally accepted definition of its function, obviously general criteria and guidelines have not yet been established. This is another reason why so little progress is being made and why the public is so uncertain about what's going on in the field.

Where does the blame go for this lack of organization and coordination? A kid gets out of medical school, serves a three-year psychiatric residency, and finally gets his license to practice headshrinking. Is it his fault that he's on his own, footloose and regulation free, from then on? There are approximately 20,000 of these guys practicing psychiatry in the U.S. today. Are they at fault as a group for floundering like fish out of water among the theories and techniques, ideologies and methodologies, groping intuitively for those they think most helpful? How can they be expected to establish acceptable patterns of procedure and to practice them nationally?

The responsibility rests, undoubtedly, with both the individual and the group. The individual psychiatrist tends to isolate himself from the psychiatric community and from the community as a whole, having as little contact as possible with other human beings. He seems to prefer his anonymity, his freedom to practice as he pleases, his lack of restraints and the necessity to answer for his mistakes. Of course, he prefers this! Isolationism, however, does not make for better psychotherapy. If anything, it paves the way for the most inferior kind of clinical practice.

The group, instead of pulling these isolated individuals together and developing some sort of professional unity, tends to support the lone god/doctor in his practice and to cover up the suspicion that this might not be achieving the best results in the treatment of mental illness. Furthermore, the group has failed to come to terms with many of the basic clinical issues involved; it has failed to lay down basic foundations, instructions, and limitations for the profession as a whole. Therefore, psychiatry is continually moving in circles, instead of forward. Pluralism may be wonderful in politics or

economics; in psychiatry it serves only to promote confusion, isolation, and despair.

The blame goes even further. How about that kid
fresh out of medical school? What kind of an education
has he been given? Has it prepared him in any special
way for a psychiatric residency? Has it even prepared
him adequately for the practice of medicine? The answer is an unqualified, no. During his residency, can the
prospective psychiatrist make up for what he didn't get
in med school? Does he leave his residency well versed
in psychotherapeutic method, confident in his knowledge
of approaches, adept at choosing the correct approach
for the individual problem? Chances again are over-
whelmingly, no.

A psychiatric resident has a variety of theories and
methods thrown at him. He latches onto first one and
then another (depending on his supervisor) as the final
answer to all problems of human behavior. At the end of
his three years, after having tasted—but never really
digested—a little bit of everything, he is left with a very
jumbled palate. No attempt is made to coordinate and
evaluate the various methods for him. No overall review
is made for him; no suggestions are given about when to
use one kind of technique or when another might work
better. Nothing is done to help him put all his concentrated learning into the proper perspective. The psychiatric resident is then thrown out into the community;
hopefully, he has some feeling of idealism for his chosen
profession, but he has little grasp of the realities involved.

Once established in the community, does he receive
any assistance from the local psychiatric association?
Local societies are made up of local psychiatrists—in
other words, several of the isolated individuals thrown
together in one room doesn't bring them out of their
isolation or make for any increased unity in the field of

psychiatry. The presentation at these meetings is usually just a hodgepodge of opinions with little attempt to validate those expressed. There is no discussion of therapies, doctor-patient relationships, the role of the psychiatrist, or the inability of so many headshrinkers to develop a warm working relationship with their patients. They certainly never discuss each other's different techniques in a meaningful way. In many instances, they don't even know what techniques they, themselves, are using.

On the national level, things are not any better. If we sent our young shrink off to an annual meeting, the most he could hope for is the superficial discussion of issues some five years overdue and maybe a cursory glance at current studies going on in the field. This much he could get from the journals, could get better by reading the literature than by sitting in a noisy, overcrowded, smoke-filled room trying to hear an author rattle off a condensed paper while fifteen other authors in other smoke-filled rooms are trying to do the same thing. With two or three hundred papers being read during the three days of an annual meeting, the result is a complete shambles. The main reason for this meeting is social; people meet people from other parts of the country and have a few drinks, as well as a tax-deductible vacation.

Psychiatry is represented by several national organizations. The largest and most influential is the American Psychiatric Association (APA) with a membership of 15,000 practicing psychiatrists, or three-quarters of the total. Perhaps the real blame for all the chaos in the field should be leveled at the APA because in over a hundred years of existence (its neophyte form can be traced back to 1844), it has never gathered its ranks together into an agreement of policies. It has never laid down a format and said, "This is psychiatry. This is what it can do; this is what it should do; and this is what it cannot do." It has

produced few, if any, able leaders and given no basic
guidance to the grassroots members looking to the
national body for positive direction.

The APA hasn't even groped with simple problems
like the ethics of practice and come up with practical,
practicable answers. If a patient is dissatisfied in some
way with a local psychiatric hospital or becomes disgruntled with a certain psychiatrist in the community—
mabe she is accusing him of making improper sexual
advances toward her—she is wasting her time to take it
up with the local psychiatric society. I don't know of a
single instance in which the Psychiatric Association
kicked somebody out because of unethical conduct. How
can the organization really condemn someone for behaving unethically when it has no definite sense of its
own identity?

Even at the present time, even in the midst of all the
confusion and frustration in the field, the APA is still
not making any effort to pull the ranks together or to
imbue them with the basic issues of psychiatry—quality
therapy, effective services, constructive research, and
prevention. Instead, the APA is currently all wrapped
up in such controversial issues as the Vietnam war, poverty, racism, youth, its income tax status, government
training grants for potential psychiatrists, and what the
topic for the next annual meeting should be. This is so
typical of the APA. It can't formulate policies about what
constitutes good psychiatric practice, but it can jump
feet first, into every other area of American concern and
come up with all kinds of out-of-thin-air advice.

A case in point is the recent poll sent to all APA members that included such magnanimous questions as:
Should we take a stand against poverty and request a revision of national priorities—less money for defense,
more for problems at home, etc? Should we take strong

stands with the legislative and administrative branches of government about contributing to the alienation of young people today? Fifty-one percent of the APA membership returned the poll, and the overall majority was in favor of taking strong stands on the issues proposed. However, just as great a majority said "yes" to the final question, "should the APA stick basically to psychiatry and not become a forum for political issues?" This was the best that the national organization of psychiatry could come up with, a poll that directly contradicted itself. The APA as a whole does not know, and its individual members can't tell you, whether it's a scientific outfit, a political organization, a social group, or just some mishmash combination of everything—where anyone can get up and shoot off his mouth and everyone else will rally round and agree or disagree. That very little of any practical value will be accomplished in the near future appears quite certain.

At the last annual meeting in San Francisco, a number of demonstrations by various liberal groups took place. The president of the APA knew this was going to happen. He had to choose among canceling the entire meeting, canceling the scientific session and devoting the meeting to a discussion of social issues, or working out some sort of compromise. He decided on the latter, admitting the groups in order to communicate with them —as if communication in itself would lead anywhere. If communication alone could solve problems, there would be no strife in the world today. It certainly didn't solve anything in this instance. The demonstrators disrupted the overall proceedings, participated in the scientific sessions, repeatedly took over the platform, and did many weird things to antagonize the members present. Consequently, our next two annual meetings are going to be devoted to alternatives to violence. As if all the headshrinkers in this country needed two years to figure out that the alternative to violence—the one and only alternative to violence—is peaceful negotiation based on mutual respect! The APA is a senile old lady trying to go up a down escalator. Its actions tend to provoke pity or anger but certainly not respect.

HOW IT ALL GOT STARTED

The current situation didn't just happen overnight. Like anything else, it has been subject to the tides of history and the tribulations of the times.

The modern era of psychiatry began approximately a hundred years ago. Prior to that time, mental patients were looked upon as freaks or devils, dangerous to themselves and society. They were locked up in dungeons and treated as animals. No attempt was made to unravel the fundamental causes of mental illness, and patients were subjected to various torture mechanisms—purging, bleeding, trephining (or drilling holes in the skull)—in order to drive out the evil spirits supposedly haunting them. Unfortunately, there are some state hospitals still in existence that haven't advanced much beyond that point.

During the nineteenth century, a widespread movement was started to humanize the treatment of mental patients. Doctors would make rounds and chat with the poor inmates, hoping in some magical way to help them. This humanistic trend, both in this country and abroad, began to undermine the centuries-old belief that mental illness was some form of devil possession. Although in and of itself it was not successful in achieving any dramatic results in the rehabilitation of patients, it did much to bring the problem of mental illness into the human and natural realm. At least it was recognized that most mental patients were not particularly destructive. Some of the chains and other forms of restraint were thrown away.

Then along came the psychoanalytic movement. The studies in hysteria by Freud and Breuer, utilizing hypnosis, were a revolutionary breakthrough in the attempt to uncover the reasons why people developed symptoms of mental illness. For the first time, doctors listened to their patients and tried to understand the nature of their conflicts. Psychoanalytic concepts, however, were so radical in relation to the thinking of the times, they had such tremendous impact and met with so much resistance from both medical and lay people, that their supporters were forced into becoming a kind of cult; Freud himself assumed the role of the messiah. From his arbitrary position of authority, Freud decided what his disciples should and should not believe. He thus preserved the movement against the storm of controversy and prevented infighting from further weakening his tenuous position.

He accepted very little deviation from his own theoretical scriptures and promptly expelled any students of the method who became original thinkers. Consequently, some very high caliber people like Adler and Jung were ostracized because their need to express themselves exceeded their need to conform to the master's teaching. This rigidity within the early psychoanalytic movement paved the way for many forms of dissent. Liberal and reform movements clashed with orthodox tradition in much the same way that such deviations struggled for power in the field of religion. Orthodox psychoanalysis, however, is on the wane and has been roundly criticized in recent years because of its isolationism and adherence to an outmoded and unscientific system of beliefs. To some extent, though, all modern psychiatry is either derived from certain aspects of psychoanalytic theory— or is a reaction to it.

The advent of the organic therapies in the 1920s and the movement to treat the mentally ill in a strictly phys- iological way ushered in the next major phase in the development of psychiatry. Early indications that mal- arial fevers were beneficial to victims of paresis (syphilis infected brains) brought about the practice of inducing high temperatures and sleep. The latter, or prolonged narcosis, was accomplished with barbiturates or gas mixtures, a practice still used with some slight success today. One thing led to another and by the midthirties, guys like Sakel, using insulin, and Von Meduna, trying first camphor in oil and then metrazol, were artificially inducing epileptic seizures that appeared to interfere with certain excitement states. In 1938 a European named Bini used electricity for the first time to stimulate convulsions, and it has been used for this purpose ever since. Simultaneous with the beginning of shock therapy was the development of psychosurgery. The Swiss had experimented with the technique toward the end of the nineteenth century, but it was Moniz and Lima in 1936 who really gave it momentum. Moniz is given credit for originating the prefrontal lobotomy.

Psychoanalysts refused to accept any part of the organic therapies, calling them throwbacks to the torture chambers of the Middle Ages. They further claimed that such methods repressed the patient's conflicts rather than brought them to light, and did more harm than good because of possible brain damage. Actually no one really knew what the various organic therapies did or why they were effective. We still don't know exactly how they work, but a number of psychiatrists, especially those frustrated by the poor results of a strictly psychoanalytic approach, continue to latch onto anything organic that might be helpful clinging to the idea that mental illness might be strictly physical after all.

The next big discovery was tranquilizers. Doctors using Phenergan to treat allergies and Rauwolfia to lower blood pressure noted the calming effects these drugs tended to have on psychotic patients. Drug companies pursued this lead and came up with various other drugs. These medications were soon making it possible for patients who had been hospitalized and completely unproductive for years to be converted into at least semiproductive, nonhospitalized citizens. And the eventual development of the less powerful tranquilizers—Meprobamate, Librium, etc. simplified the treatment of less severe mental ailments. This new approach gave added impetus to the physiological movement going on within psychiatry, and more headshrinkers tended to become medically oriented in the treatment of their patients. They would prescribe one type of tranquilizer for the neurotic patient, an antidepressant for the depressed patient, another medication for the schizophrenic, etc.

Analysts again levied their objections. They argued that tranquilizers covered up the patient's conflicts rather than resolved them. Excited and anxious patients merely became zombies on the drugs, and occasionally the side effects were fatal, so what the hell good were they, anyway? Such objections, however, ignored the fact that tranquilizers were enabling hospitals to reduce their census considerably. Psychoanalysis has never been effective treatment for schizophrenic or acutely psychotic patients.

Maybe the patients were not really cured by the drugs, but they did get over the acute phase of the illness faster and could go home sooner.

The most recent development is the trend toward community mental health centers to bring treatment to the masses. This became a joint effort of the government and the news media when the shocking truth leaked out of some state hospitals that patients were dying and remained undiscovered for several days. About this time President Kennedy, who had a built-in interest in mental health because of a retarded sister, took office and gave the movement his full administrative support. The basic idea was to provide psychiatric services to all victims of psychiatric disturbances who needed them. It was also an attempt to provide patients with neighborhood treatment facilities, theoretically allowing them to be rehabilitated in terms of family and community, rather than shipping them off to distant hospitals and treating them as socially isolated individuals. Psychiatrists, too, gave this movement full support until many of them began realizing that quality of care was being sacrificed for quantity.

Right now we are in what might be called the "do your own thing" phase. Books are being published that describe anywhere from twenty to one hundred different psychiatric approaches to human problems. It's not enough, for example, to talk about group therapy anymore. You now have to specify whether it's a T-group, an encounter group, a family therapy group, a couple's group, a gestalt therapy group, or a group to learn about group therapy. Nonmedical treatment centers are springing up everywhere, such as the Esalen weekend retreats in California, the Recovery Inc. meetings, Neurotics Anonymous, and the screamingly amateurish sensitivity confrontations in every other church basement. The ancillary professions (psychology and social work) are getting in on the act, and all sorts of hair-brained techniques are being pressed into service. Patients are being deconditioned and desensitized, when they are not being reconditioned and resensitized, by a host of semiskilled professionals and unskilled laymen, each of whom is "doing his own thing." Even the witch doctors are being reincarnated to help certain minority groups. The public must be as totally bewildered as I am, and I'm supposed to be able to comprehend all this nonsense! Current attitudes toward psychiatry vary all the way from loving to despising it. And in between are those who feel it's okay if you really need it, those who feel it's some kind of evil engendered by the fast pace of modern life, and those who are highly skeptical about anything even remotely related to the field.

To put it on the line: (1) Psychiatry does have a very valid function to perform in our society. (2) The organic therapies are out except in specialized situations and extreme cases. (3) Tranquilizers have their place, but without competent psychiatric supervision of their use, they are worse than useless. (4) Psychoanalysis as a separate, isolated institution can no longer survive. (5) The community psychiatric movement, although it has succeeded in bringing psychiatric facilities closer to the patient, has not followed up with sufficient treatment in depth; the average patient going to the typical clinic has no assurance that he will receive the treatment he needs. (6) The "do your own thing" phase of psychiatry has only served to further obfuscate the issues involved with the result that each psychiatrist is going off on his own tangent with little objective basis for the kind of therapy he practices. All in all, there is no accountability for treatment or results, and whether a patient goes to a public or private facility, he is at the mercy of people who quite possibly don't know a damn thing about what they're doing or why they are doing it. That's a pretty sordid indictment of my own profession, but that's the way it has been for the last hundred years.

WHAT'S CAUSING THE CURRENT CRISIS?

I began this chapter by pointing out that a helluva lot of money is being swept into the mainstream of mental health services with very little to show for it. I went on to criticize the field for having no specific standard for measuring its strengths and weaknesses, the value of its clinical methods, or the amount of its therapeutic success. One of the greatest obstacles in the development and practice of psychiatry today is its inability to quantify results in a strictly scientific fashion. Even more disenchanting is the fact that psychiatry may never be able to measure itself accurately or function within a purely deductive frame of reference.

It's all a question of epistemology, really. Epistemology is a philosophical term referring to the roots of human knowledge—where it comes from and how you go about getting it. As far as nineteenth- and twentieth-century man is concerned, scientific method is the answer, the whole answer. When it comes to observing human behavior, however, and the whole area of motivation, when it comes to why people do things to themselves and to other people, why they have the feelings they have, why they lose touch with the real world and invent imaginary worlds of their own, why they destroy themselves with drugs and booze, why they are anxious or fearful or compulsive, then you're in a whole different realm, and scientific method is useless, or at best of only limited utility. When a person tells me he feels depressed, he has to use words and that alone gives the situation a subjective rather than objective climate. Furthermore, I can't suddenly pull out a little gadget and say, "Okay, let's measure the amount of depression you feel." Even if I could, it wouldn't mean anything. There are thousands of different human emotions and different gradations of them, and there is just no way of evaluating them, either on a mass basis or on the individual level. What causes severe depression in one person might not distress another person at all. Saying that such and such an amount of depression causes such and such a degree of pathology or illness in the normal person is as meaningless as saying the sky is blue. As a matter of fact, we're not even sure what "normality" is supposed to be.

The crucial problem facing psychiatry, then, is not just that there is no such thing in existence as a total theory of human behavior, one which embraces all facets of human interaction and all aspects of scientific method, one which promotes the formulation of hypotheses and their testing in new contexts, as is possible in fields such as physics and chemistry. The crucial problem is that there probably never will be such a theory! The same problem exists in sociology and psychology. In the realm of human behavior it's every man for himself. You can construct theories of personality and theories of mental function. You can even go along with the latest attempts to relate different systems of interaction to each other in a meaningful way, thinking along computer lines and psychocybernetics; but no one of these formulations encompasses all human behavior, nor can any of them be successfully adapted to rigorous scientific testing. As a result, psychiatry is right back where it started. It is lost in a quagmire of different theories and approaches, none of which does justice to all of the observable facts or all of the different situations that human beings find themselves in. Of course such a situation is causing a crisis!

The second problem shaking up the field is a direct outgrowth of the first. Many shrinks, erroneously assuming that psychiatry is an exact science in the sense of physics and chemistry, attempt to extrapolate from their knowledge of psychopathology to all existing human situations—social, religious, political, economic, the works. They are overextending themselves into areas where they have no competency.

The psychiatrist is supposed to treat individual disturbances, not take on society's problems as a whole. This problem may appear to have a simple solution— curtail all activity not immediately within psychiatry's sphere. Psychiatrists, however, are inextricably involved in many other areas and, in order to be effective in treating individuals, must be wrapped up in those problems affecting the population as a whole. Take the welfare system, for example. A psychiatrist treating a patient for depression may discover that poverty factors are contributing significantly to the condition. Until these factors are licked, he's just spinning his wheels as far as trying to erase the depression. He's in a position, therefore, to go to the welfare department and say, "Look, one of the reasons this patient is so sick is that he's so poor. He needs help from you people now." Unfortunately, the welfare system in this country is so fixated on it's own ways of doing things that it doesn't lend itself well to working in an interdisciplinary fashion with other fields. (In this case, for example, the welfare supervisor might accept the psychiatrist's recommendation for a telephone but refuse to appropriate a thousand dollars to put a new roof on the house.) As a result, the psychiatrist's role is necessarily and immediately expanded to cover the problems of welfare as well as those of his own clinical practice. This can't be prevented entirely, and it would probably be a mistake to try. Psychiatrists, in one way or another, do have to serve as consultants to various social agencies in the community, but not at the expense of their primary job, which is treating patients in the clinical situation.

The legal field is another attractive playground. Psychiatrists are frequently called into the courtroom to attest to an individual's sanity—a game that's so meaningless it's a farce. One shrink gets on the stand and "proves" the prisoner totally insane; the second one gets up with his battery of test results and "proves" him totally sane. Our legal system presupposes that the truth about human behavior is either black or white. Psychiatry presupposes that it's *never* black or white. You cannot mix these two approaches using the adversary system. It has to be done with some extralegal format that doesn't exist at the present time. It might never exist if psychiatry suddenly withdraws from the system. The fact of the matter is that psychiatry cannot withdraw, but it can be better confined to its area of expertise.

The relationship between religion and psychiatry is another big problem. A minister once told me that he would never recommend psychiatry because its practitioners were all atheists. Number one, all psychiatrists are not atheists and, number two, their religious views have no relevance to their patient's problems. As a resident, I was told never to get involved in a patient's religious hang-ups; if a clergyman called me in reference to a particular case, I was to refuse to discuss the matter with him. At the other end are those shrinks who are forever speaking to church groups about psychiatry and religion as if psychiatry had all the answers on religious issues. Somewhere in between these extremes is the fact that psychiatry does have something relevant to say about those religious views contributing to human psychopathology. There are certain pathological religious

beliefs being handed down from generation to generation—the doctrine of original sin for one—and these beliefs should be the real concern of psychiatrists. Such
issues are seldom discussed in public. When invited to
address the members of a specific religious denomina-
tion, the psychiatrist avoids the main sources of conflict
for fear of alienating a whole segment of the community.

I have already alluded to the politics of psychiatry.
Unfortunately, the politics of psychiatry are just as superficial and desultory as the politics of politics. The people
who get into positions of power within the psychiatric
associations are usually those people who enjoy power
for its own sake. They grab hold of an issue that happens
to be in favor, hop on the bandwagon, develop lobby
groups, and try to get legislation passed—all for the sake
of political aspirations rather than promoting quality
of care. Community mental health is a good illustration.
Most officers of psychiatric associations don't know how
to deliver adequate mental health services to anyone,
much less to everyone. When mental health for the masses gained national recognition and became a federal
campaign issue, our psychiatric associations rallied to
the call and gave it their full support primarily to enhance their own images in the community.

A current APA concern is how to become more
involved in politics without becoming a political organization. At the present time, many national professional
associations enjoy a tax-exempt status. However, if their
basic reason for being turns out to be political, they
lose this status. This has already happened to the American Medical Association (AMA), but it has gotten around
it somewhat by forming a secondary organization called
AMPAC. While separate from the AMA, AMPAC's sole
purpose is to express AMA political policies. Now the
APA is wondering if it should form its own little political

satellite or join forces with the AMA's. I'm sure this question will be paramount in forthcoming APA conventions.

Here again, politics should not be a primary concern of the psychiatrist, yet psychiatry does need to be involved. Psychiatric associations do need political representation, not on the basis of political faddism the way it is today (delivery of care versus the kind of care delivered) but on the basis of the issues that are relevant to the mental health of the population. If psychiatry doesn't maintain a voice in Washington, it will lose control of the legislative measures relating to it, measures such as those now being considered by Congress on drug abuse, alcoholism, and national health care. In addition, it will have to relinquish the administration of these programs to people outside the field who have no more basis for telling psychiatrists how to run their business than psychiatrists have for telling them how to run theirs. If psychiatry limits itself to the simple provision of services to the sick and washes its hands of the more complex roles of legislation and prevention, it is merely shoveling sand against the tide and its effectiveness will eventually be washed away entirely. In other words, in all these different areas, it's not a matter of whether psychiatry should or should not extend itself, but how far it should go. This question only the field itself can answer—if it ever gets around to it.

A third problem contributing to the crisis is the lack of decent research in the field and the resulting poor literature. The scarcity of good basic research, despite the millions being spent, is appalling. That's a tremendous indictment of any endeavor, but it spells suicide in a young, raw field like psychiatry, straining at its very core for growth and recognition. Psychiatry must progress to survive, but it cannot possibly do so without sound, basic, intensive research.

At the moment, the two bulwarks holding up production in research are the federal government and psychiatry, itself. Private research funds have virtually dried up
as far as psychiatry or medical research is concerned.
The government took over that function when it established the National Institutes of Health, including the
National Institute of Mental Health, and has concentrated largely on methodology rather than on substance.
A subjective field like psychiatry, as much an art as a
science, just doesn't lend itself to dissection and rigid
postulates. It goes back to that same hang-up on scientific method. Scientific method consists of two approaches,
deductive and inductive. Using the deductive approach,
the researcher projects a hypothesis, experiments and
collects data accordingly, and decides if the hypothesis
is valid. The inductive researcher does his observing and
collects his data first and then draws his conclusions.
Although both practices are acceptable, deductive research is far more prevalent than inductive and is the
only kind smiled upon by Uncle Sam.

Getting research money out of the government
depends not so much on how brilliant you are or how
adept you are at probing the depths of the unknown, but
on how well you can reduce the area of study to a pseudo-
scientific format—developing ways of organizing the
material, accounting in advance for all materials, and
forecasting the probable results. Your prime dedication
must be to filling out forms! The man who applies for a
research grant today, saying that he doesn't know too
much about the problems he is approaching or how to
tackle them in a systematic fashion but that he wants to
collect some hard data and then develop a theory that
seems meaningful in light of the data, wouldn't have a
chance. As a matter of fact, Freud himself wouldn't have

a prayer. His efforts to develop a body of knowledge and organize it in a meaningful way were purely inductive; he listened to his patients, analyzed what they said, and then constructed his hypotheses. In other words, if you're a good psychiatrist you're licked before you start. You're automatically prevented from doing good psychiatric research for the same reasons that you can't adapt formal measurements and statistics to the clinical practice of psychiatry.

On the other hand, you're also prevented from carrying out good studies by your own associates. Most shrinks are so insecure in their profession and so self-conscious that they won't allow themselves to be audited or monitored in any way. They can think up a thousand different reasons as to why auditing would interfere with their work. Even resident psychiatrists, still in training pants, are sensitive about this, and when I was conducting a residency program I had a helluva time with some of them when I brought in a video-tape recorder for the purpose of observing their work. This, of course, eliminates any line of productive research on what good psychotherapy is all about. It eliminates the empirical basis for finding out what constitutes good clinical practice. It virtually slams the door in the face of any major improvement in psychotherapy. In a multimillion dollar project, the Menninger Institute has been trying to find out whether psychotherapy actually helps anyone. The pertinent question is how the good therapist manages to produce consistent positive results and what distinguishes his work from that of his less competent associates. Because of the way research funds are being appropriated today, because of the misunderstood or mistaken variables concerned, conclusions—if any are ever reached—have been few and far between.

If research in the field is bad, the literature is even worse. It's only logical that bad studies are going to yield bad reports, and a glance through any of the psychiatric journals more than bears this out. I picked up a recent one at random to corroborate what I'm saying and discovered such gems as "The Destructive Potential of Humor in Psychotherapy," "Observations on Suicidal Behavior in Indians," "Lithium in Pregnancy," and "Training Police in Community Relations."

The article on humor (written, incidentally, by one of our more distinguished psychiatrists) suggests that while humor has its place in life, it is of limited value in the therapeutic situation. On the contrary, I have found humor to be one of the most forceful weapons in the arsenal of the therapist, one that, when used properly, can turn an apparently untreatable patient into a treatable one. What this most distinguished psychiatrist should have done was to investigate ways of using humor to promote better psychotherapy rather than discouraging its use because of possible repercussions.

The suicide-in-Indians study is an NIMH production. It points out that the breakdown of traditional values and widespread unemployment on our reservations are significant sociocultural factors in producing the higher suicide rates among American Indians. These little tidbits of knowledge have been known for years. The Center for Studies of Suicide Prevention at NIMH must be at the bottom of the barrel if this is the best it can offer professionals trying to prevent suicide, much less Indians who are prone to it. A classic indication of psychiatry's research and literary bankruptcy is its seemingly compulsive need to reduplicate studies that have already been done, and in much greater depth, by qualified people in other fields.

The authors of "Lithium in Pregnancy" report the conflicting evidence of lithium's harmful effects and detail six precautions in its use during pregnancy. They neglect to point out (because if they did, there would have been no reason to write the article) that lithium has not been proven useful as a psychotropic drug, that it doesn't accomplish any more than other less toxic tranquilizers, and that its use, therefore, during pregnancy or at any other time is superfluous. The fact that its use must be accompanied by routine, expensive laboratory tests also does not seem to deter these authors.

The article on training police in community relations and urban problems attempts to redefine law enforcement agencies as a vital bridge between community problems and psychiatric service. Our police forces have already been acting in this capacity for years, and I could only wonder, in this instance, if the authors had familiarized themselves with the classic study by Bard and Berkowitz on training local patrolmen as specialists in family crisis intervention. The latter authors were successful because they had both served with the police force and really knew what they were talking about.

To make a long story short, for every constructive psychiatric article published, there are approximately a thousand that are useless. When you consider how many journals there are today in the field of mental health and how much money is being spent by the NIMH on phony research projects, the figures are frightening. Most of the research currently being done in the field is a complete waste of time, money, and energy because it is too limited in scope, too faulty in design, and not correlated well enough with what we already know.

There are other major hassles in psychiatry. The paucity of good training facilities, a part of the poor system of education, is one. The real problem of class-cultural differences is another. The fact that psychiatry remains but a stepchild of medicine is still another. The horrendous variety of approaches and the previously mentioned difficulty of systematizing psychiatry as a body of knowledge is a very basic problem, tied in with a lot of the hang-ups I have already cited. The diagnostic problem, or problem of illness classification, goes along with all this, as does the apparent elusiveness of psychiatric truth.

There are minor difficulties such as the lack of good cooperation between psychiatry and the ancillary professions, the failure of many insurance companies to cover mental illness, the ineffectiveness of self-policing, the gross manpower shortage, and the ever present communication gap among psychiatrists themselves.

With so many unsolved and unsolvable problems of its own, you are probably wondering what right psychiatry has to hang out a shingle, much less assume that it can cope with you and your problems. In many cases, you're quite wise in challenging the field. At this writing, there very definitely is a lot of second-rate psychotherapy being spieled out to you, the gullible consumer, the guy with dollars in his pocket and desperation in his soul. Competent psychiatry, however scarce it may be, does exist in this country. The competent psychiatrist does prove, over and over, his ingenious capacity to deal with life's basic problems, to take the depressed and the neurotic, the suicidal and the psychotic, the unsociable and the addicted by the hand and lead them back into the bosom of society and the warmth of their own worthiness, back into the land of the living and the happy to be alive. Therein lies a glimmer of redemption. Despite all shortcomings, the field of psychiatry contains within its ranks some men who have mastered their field despite the billion dollar blunderbuss that masquerades as psychiatry today.

CHAPTER **2**

Will The Real Psychiatrist
Please Stand Up

"WHY THE HELL would anyone want to go into psychiatry?" my father snorted when I told him at the end of my first year in medical school that was my choice. His attitude was typical of parents whose sons are studying to become doctors. They want them all to study surgery. They seem to think that unless you're out there dramatically pulling people through last minute operations, you're not doing that much. You're missing all the glamor of medicine. As far as my father was concerned, psychiatry not only wasn't surgery, it wasn't even a bona fide member of the medical hierarchy.

There are a number of reasons why doctors go on to psychiatry. Some have problems themselves and are looking for answers. Others have a kind of scoptophilia, or a desire to see and hear about other people's sex lives. Still others are forced into it because they're neither bright enough nor energetic enough to go into one of the other specialties. Many are bribed into it by government grants. A proportionately large number of Jews go the headshrinking route because it's one of few disciplines where they can find a sense of identity and common bond with other human beings in an essentially Gentile world. Probably the vast majority of young shrinks enter the field out of a subconscious fear of losing control of their emotions. This hasn't been proven, although research has established that a great many doctors go into medicine because of a fear of death. I suspect it's also a powerful motivator in pulling certain types one step further into a psychiatric specialty. This would partially explain why so many shrinks are emotionally flat, lack spontaneity, and are distant in their relations with others. They overcontrol for fear of losing control.

Doctors as a professional group appear to have more problems than other professional groups; the suicide rate is certainly higher in the medical profession and highest of all among psychiatrists! This is probably a result of their isolating themselves so much from their own humanity. A competent psychiatrist learns to integrate his own feelings and emotions, his own humanity, with those of his patients. Few psychiatrists, however, are really competent and consequently, very few are able to do this. Because of the tenuousness of the field and the rather shaky images they have of themselves, most psychiatrists instead feel they must hide behind some facade or veneer of professionalism and deny their right to be just ordinary human beings. Many of them even have the ridiculous idea that they must set themselves up as gods in order to practice successful psychotherapy. Some eventually isolate themselves so completely from the human race, even from their own families, that they have nothing left to live for and they disentegrate.

When psychiatrists do crack up, man, they go all the way—drugs, drinking, and finally suicide. They're extremely hard to treat because their fantasy for so long has been that they're the ones with all the answers. They're God. Who does God go to for treatment? Other psychiatrists are reluctant to treat them. Somehow it is a reflection on themselves. When a shrink cracks up and the rest of us recognize and deal with it as we would with any other patient, that means we're all just human beings after all. Heaven forbid that we openly recognize this fact and blow to bits some of the silly little fantasies that dominate the psychiatric scene! But to become a good psychiatrist, that's precisely what you have to do. To become a really capable psychotherapist, you first have to become a well-rounded, well-adjusted, sensitive, secure, self-aware human being.

I went into psychiatry because I was more interested in improving the quality of human life than I was in promoting longevity. As a kid I had toyed with the idea of going into cancer research and looking for ways to prolong human life. After watching many people drag on year after year in a semiexistence, not because of physical illness but because of emotional problems that kept them constantly stirred up, I began to realize that the number of years a person lived was not nearly so important as how he spent those years. Born during the depression and on the wrong side of town, I was a daily witness not only to man's inhumanity toward man but also to the ways in which people made themselves even more miserable than they really had to be. I promised myself that if there were only some way, some magical way to reconcile their differences and make their lives more productive, I would find it.

As I grew older, I could see that what was going on in my own little corner correlated with what was going

on in the world at large. Although science had extended
the average lifetime some thirty years, it hadn't done
much to make those extra years worth living. The Korean
thing had hit the fan and was just as controversial as
Vietnam. People were starving in all parts of the world.
Oppressed minority groups and ghettos were everywhere,
not just on my block; divorce was widespread; parents
were mutilating children; old people were rotting away
in institutions, forgotten. I thought by becoming a psychiatrist, I could right some of these wrongs. I could get
down to the ground level of human behavior, its motiva-
tions and aberrations, and find out why it seemed so
self-destructive. Then I realized what a paradox the
doctor's role was in society. His function is a direct anti-
thesis to his dedication—he is expected to patch people
up just so society can destroy them again in one way
or another. My doubts about the strictly physical side
of medicine were confirmed. It looked as if men's minds
needed healing more than their bodies.

Once convinced that a purely medical, or scientific,
route was not the answer, I knocked off my premed
courses in a hurry and spent the rest of my time as an
undergraduate in liberal arts. I delved into philosophy,
which started me questioning the nature of man himself,
the great contrast between capabilities and actual performance. Sociology showed me that there was a contra-
diction in society, too, that it was not operating for
its own betterment. I remember reading an article by
Albert Einstein in which he attempted to relate ethical
principles to a scientific methodology, and becoming
intensely interested in his idea that underneath everything—science, the humanities, all human function—was
some sort of aesthetic principle. Here was the foremost
scientist of our times also expressing dissatisfaction with
man and society and concerning himself with things of

value in human life, saying that somehow ways could be found to improve the human situation, that science and the humanities could be brought into one focus for the betterment of mankind.

I was terribly impressed by Einstein's proposal. I became absorbed with the notion of applying the scientific method, not in the rigid narrow-sense way it's taught in school but more in the inductive sense as Einstein did using intuition to find answers, to make assumptions, and then to find out how to prove them in the real world. In my youthful enthusiasm, it actually seemed possible to create an ideal society by using inductive reasoning, to end war, for instance, by setting up several hypotheses and trying first one and then another until the right combination came along. I still think a great deal could be accomplished if more effort were made in intellectual and educational circles to unite the two disciplines, to look for ways in which they complement each other rather than to stress their dissimilarities continually. Until we discover all the angles, however, until we know how to make scientific method work for the humanities and vice versa, we have to compromise—and to me, psychiatry seemed like the most promising solution.

As if I didn't have enough on my mind at the time, I fell for a narcissistic little creature who was very appealing physically but had so many emotional hang-ups I never knew what to expect next. I dangled on her string for several months before finally realizing how naïve I was in this whole area of male/female relationships. This. on top of my first year of medical school, which is about the worst thing that could happen to anyone, wiped out any lingering ambitions I might have held for straight medicine and convinced me completely that psychiatry was the place for me, the only place.

I don't think I ever convinced my father, however. He never did develop an appreciation for the attributes of psychiatry but from time to time would ask derogatory questions like, "What's all this psychiatry stuff about anyway?" and "Do you ever cure anyone?" To him, being a psychiatrist was the same thing as being a welfare worker—passing out food stamps to people who couldn't afford to eat. Well, in some ways, he was probably right. In other ways, though, he was dead wrong.

IN THE MAKING

It's one thing to decide to go into psychiatry, quite another to become a psychiatrist. All persons practicing psychotherapy in the United States today are not graduate psychiatrists. The laws in most states regulating this sort of thing are less than strict or totally nonexistent. Virtually anyone, whether qualified, educated, experienced, or not, can offer his services as a marriage counselor, family planner, analyst, spiritualist, advisor, or anything that strikes his fancy and brings in the bread. If properly trained and regulated, some of these people could probably be very helpful in the general field of mental health. But right now, with everybody getting into the act, from cousin Genevieve who had a couple of divorces herself and bases her "counseling" on "experience," to that funny old man who passes out those weird religious tracts, the public must be wary.

Accredited people, besides psychiatrists, in the mental health field are social workers, psychiatric nurses, psychologists, and a few lay psychoanalysts. These people have received fairly standardized courses of training and are considered qualified; some of them may even be competent.

Psychiatrists must first become medical doctors, then go on to specialize in psychiatry. The present requirements include four years of premed, four years of medical school, a year of internship, three years of residency, and a lifetime of frustration and elucidation. This is not a particularly good system for producing qualified psychiatrists, far from it, but fortunately there are movements afoot to change the existing curriculum. The medical manpower shortage alone is enough to make the government and other concerned parties start hollering for fewer eggheads and more clinicians. Anyone who has been through the twelve-year mill knows that not only would a constructive revision of the system produce more doctors, but would give us more qualified specialists in a shorter period of time.

As it stands now, the four years of medical school are almost a complete waste of time. Although some schools are finally getting away from so much irrelevant lab work, a lot of them still devote the first year to the dissection and anatomy of the human body, rote memorization of the tendons, ligaments, muscles, veins, arteries, nerves, etc.—all things that are largely unrelated to developing skill as a physician.

My first year of medical school was spent with a two-hundred pound female cadaver, copies of Morris' *Anatomy* and Cunningham's *Dissection Manual*, and a sadistic little professor who didn't believe in answering questions but shouted, "Look it up. The answers are all in the book." every time a baffled student approached him. I was supposed to uncover such things as the mysteries of the digestive tract, the maze of the respiratory system, the relationship between the liver and the spleen and a whole lot more, but half the time I didn't have the vaguest notion about what I was cutting up and trying to examine. I wasn't even certain I would be finishing the course, much less three more years of med school, because halfway through I became so disgruntled with the whole setup that I wrote the professor a letter criticizing his course and his teaching methods. It took them quite a while to decide whether or not that made me unfit for the medical profession. Before I got out of that mess, I rubbed opinions with the dean and several heads of departments and ended up repeating the damn anatomy course. The only thing I learned the second time around that I hadn't learned the first, was to keep my big mouth shut.

The second year is spent in the lab, staring through a microscope at bits of feces to see if they contain parasites. First of all, that's a lab technician's job. Second, pathologists are the only doctors who need to become expert in this area. And third, what the hell good is it going to do a psychiatrist to be able to recognize intestinal parasites? The final two years are a little more productive; they at least introduce you to the clinical situation; during the last year, you actually get to work on patients. I even got a taste of psychiatry that fourth year, a once-a-week lecture parroting the textbooks and an occasional chance to interview psychiatric patients under the supervision of a psychiatrist. Otherwise, my four years of med school contributed little or nothing toward my professional development. If anything, they were negative in this sense, so negative they probably turned some people off who might eventually have also gone into the field.

Were medical school curriculums to become more oriented to particular branches of medicine, students could be taught everything they need to know in considerably less than four years. Right now, the programs are limited to a little physiology, biochemistry, pathology, and anatomy—all rather irrelevant to the practice of good medicine, certainly to the practice of a specialty like psychiatry. What they should be emphasizing is the correlation of structure with function (especially disordered function), showing students how to correlate physiology with anatomy and clinical practice so the whole pattern fits together better. Medical students need some good clinics in medicine, need to know what goes on in surgery, need to see a little obstetrics.

Potential psychiatrists need courses in the organic diseases that mimic and are associated with true psychiatric illness. If changes were made in the curriculum, these same students could be given a common foundation for any medical specialty in two or three years. They could specialize for another two or three years, practice a couple of years following that in a supervised setting, and finally be ready to go out on their own within six to eight years as opposed to twelve or more. They would be better clinicians on top of it. In addition, a more efficient educational system would enable medical schools to turn out more medical assistants as well, a trend that has proven worthwhile in European countries for generations and that would further alleviate the manpower shortage over here.

I had now spent eight years studying to become a headshrinker and still didn't know the first thing about treating mental illness. During the ninth year I did a rotating internship at Los Angeles County General Hospital, delivered babies for several weeks, fixed hernias for a while, and finally got a taste of what mental illness was really all about when I spent six weeks at the psychiatric unit, a disposal center for the whole Los Angeles area. The hospital retained the few patients it thought it could help, but channeled the large majority into state hospitals. That was like saying to nine out of ten patients who came through their doors that nothing could be done for them, and they would have to spend an indefinite period of time in an institution. To an eager, sensitive, uninitiated intern, this situation was highly depressing, but I accepted it as a challenge. I was young, idealistic, and enthusiastic; I didn't care how many problems existed or how elusive the answers were. I was going to do something about them and was going to practice competent psychiatry in spite of them. What I didn't realize was how long it was going to take me to learn how to practice good psychiatry or to figure out what the hell was really going on in the field.

By definition, the purpose of an approved psychiatric residency training program is to expose students to as many methods and approaches as possible. Never mind how confused the poor guys become or how many tangents they go off on. Just shove it at them and hope in the end they will somehow have it all organized and systematized in the best possible way for treating patients, even though the field as a whole hasn't been able to do this. One of the biggest drawbacks in these programs is the students themselves. Most of them come from middle- or upper-class, white, Anglo-Saxon, Protestant, or Jewish backgrounds. On the other hand, many mentally ill patients come from the lower-income group and the more oppressed minority groups. A psychiatrist's education really begins in the cradle, and he brings to his practice the accumulation of a lifetime's experiences with people; the fact that he relates best with those of the middle class, those who in a way are least in need of his services, is more a hindrance than an asset. The field desperately needs representation from more classes of people. It needs Negroes. It needs Indians. It needs women. It needs Mexicans and Puerto Ricans, Catholics and Quakers. It needs poor as well as rich guys, people who can come down off their theoretical pedestals and

talk to the fellow next door about his troubles. With so
many middle-class people already in the field, and having already assumed those positions of power that govern
the grants and the acceptances, the tendency is toward
even more middle-class people getting in. A kid out of
the ghetto has to make it on brains and brawn; he struggles just to gain entry into the system. A kid from the
suburbs makes it just by being from the suburbs; he
struggles for power within the system.

I wanted to see psychiatry on all levels so I divided
my three years of residency among a state hospital, a
VA hospital, and a private hospital. With the arrival of tranquilizers and crisis intervention techniques, patients in
mental hospitals are calmed down, at least outwardly,
and do not exhibit extreme symptoms of their mental
diseases. In fact, with more and more patients qualify-
ing for third-party payment and receiving private care,
it is becoming increasingly difficult to find good clinical
material for students to work on. But our state hospitals
used to be museums of psychopathology, and the Wor-
cester State Hospital in all its medieval armor, was still
going strong when I arrived. It took me fifteen minutes,
climbing stairways and slipping through locked doors,
just to get from the hospital's front entrance to my ward.
When I did arrive, it was to come face to face with a room
full of zombies; long-term, hard-core, chronically ill
schizophrenics and brain-damaged people who had been
there for years and were virtually at the end of the road.
Mental illness is like physical illness in that the longer
it goes untreated, the harder it is to treat. These poor
souls had been there so long without receiving any real
treatment that it was next to impossible to find even one
who could be interviewed in depth. My supervisor,
a psychoanalyst and a brilliant guy, if a sonofabitch,
was getting me all excited about the usefulness of

psychoanalytic technique, but there was no one around to use it on. It had virtually no application to the inpatients I was seeing at that time, and very little to the few outpatients coming back to the hospital for therapy. His intellectual formulations somehow didn't apply to the emotional problems of my patients. I ended up getting a lot of theoretical information but not much practical knowhow.

The following year I went over to the Boston VA Hospital where they were teaching a technique of applied psychoanalysis, making a form of psychotherapy out of it in what appeared to be a sensible way. They used tape recordings of actual sessions with patients, allowing residents to listen to the interchange between therapist and patient and explaining in detail why certain things were said and what reactions they elicited from the patient. They provided us with a ward full of neurotics, who could be used as teaching cases, and followed through with seminars that included discussions, demonstrations, and more tapes. It was the perfect teaching setup, and again, it was very stimulating mentally. On the practical level, however, there just weren't that many patients to whom psychoanalytic techniques could be applied directly or even indirectly, the way they were suggesting they could.

By now I was really frustrated. I was an avid reader and in the abstract probably knew as much as anyone about the various theories, especially psychoanalysis. Yet, I still couldn't make them work in the clinical situation, couldn't treat patients satisfactorily. I was constantly getting hung up on the practical applications. This time I went over to McLean Hospital which had the best inpatient setup I could find, and which concentrated on intensive treatment of acutely psychotic patients. I became heavily involved in the twenty-four-hour-a-day milieu therapy in which all aspects of the environment are controlled, and in trying to find out just how far you can go with acutely psychotic patients if you really want to knock yourself out. This time also I had plenty of patients to work with, but I was still dissatisfied. Most of them did not get well quickly, as I thought they might. I found we frequently prolonged illnesses by endeavoring to solve all of the emotional problems at once, before the patients were psychologically prepared to deal with them. Little attention was paid to how long patients stayed in the hospital as long as they could afford to stay.

Following McLean, I went into the Army for two years; again I dealt mostly with acute psychotics but this time I relied heavily, following the Army's custom, on shock therapy and tranquilizers. The Army wants to get patients out and home as soon as possible so it convulses the recent memories out of them and sends thm on their way, not really cured but probably without acute symptoms. Hopefully somebody at their local VA hospital will then take over with more intensive therapy (but I wouldn't count on it). The shrinks I met in uniform as part of the regular Army were often more in need of treatment than the cases coming in off the front lines.

Finally I made the last formal move toward becoming a recognized psychiatrist—I passed the exams given by the American Board of Psychiatry and Neurology. This made me "board certified." No psychiatrist actually requires this stamp of approval in order to practice. He does have to pass the regular M.D. exams but only certain administrative and teaching jobs demand that he also pass the psychiatry boards. I can't recall the last time a patient asked me whether or not I was board certified. Most people are simply not aware of the fact that this is the establishment's last-ditch, feeble effort to separate the wheat from the chaff among psychiatrists.

Knowing this, however, will not in itself better enable
you to find a competent shrink.

It had now been fourteen years since I signed up for
that first course in premed. I was married, had two kids
and was beginning to sport a receding hairline. For all
intents and purposes, I was ready to hang out my shingle
and begin curing the world of its mental and emotional
ills—still the most debilitating as far as I could see. The
only trouble was I didn't really know very much about
how to do it! Fourteen years and I was in just as much of
a muddle as I was way back in undergraduate school. I
still had all those unanswered questions about science
versus human behavior. I still hand't mastered the whole
spectrum of male/female relationships. I still didn't
know when to use what approach on which patient or
why certain techniques made some people worse. The
only thing I was sure of was my utter need to acquire a
much deeper, much more practical, much more comprehensive understanding of the whole field.

I tried private practice awhile, setting up a small
office in San Antonio when I got out of service. Although
patients didn't complain much, my experiences with
them just confirmed how unprepared I was. I basically
had two quandries. Some patients were getting well too
fast, before I had a chance to delve into all their underlying conflicts and apply all my painfully acquired theoretical knowledge; I felt cheated. Other patients weren't
getting well at all—despite my brilliance and versatility.
I used a lot of methods including psychoanalytic psychotherapy, interpersonal relationship therapy, reality
therapy, medication, etc. I still was never certain why
some of it succeeded and some of it didn't. I refused to
fall back on all the old psychiatric clichés like "the
patient isn't motivated for treatment," or "he's fixated
at a pregenital level of development," or "she has

regressed to a very infantile state and all you can do is wait until she decides to grow up." I considered these explanations to be mere rationalizations for poor results. There had to be a better way. Sure I was frustrated and impatient, but I could not accept these phony excuses.

I decided I had better get back into a situation that would lend itself to my further professional growth. I was convinced that my residency hadn't prepared me adequately to practice psychotherapy and that certain basic ingredients had been left out of those fourteen years despite the fact that the establishment had given me its final blessing. After looking around, I hit on the midwest. There, psychiatric circles are less rigid and more open minded, offering more of a growth situation than the east or west coasts. I settled in Milwaukee where I headed up a psychosomatic type of clinic and did some teaching. Psychosomatics intrigued me because it went back to that same old idea of relating mental and physical processes; I felt that the clue to all my unanswered questions might lie in this particular area. I remained in Milwaukee seven years, combining the traditional role of physician with that of headshrinker, using knowledge from both fields to investigate symptoms and treat patients. Finally, things began falling into place for me.

I dabbled with research. I involved myself in community problems. I got into public mental health and tangled with the bureaucracy. I also attended an annual forum brought about to integrate community psychiatry and education (at the time I was directing a residency program myself). For the first time I really began to put it all together. I learned how to adapt individual techniques to individual patients. I learned that you have to help the acute patient recover from his illness and put his life in order before you can tackle his underlying conflicts. I found out that you deal only with those things you have to deal with in order to accomplish the first goal first. I discovered how to relate to patients, all kinds of patients from all varieties of backgrounds. Most of all, I learned how to look for the relevant issues. A psychiatrist can go off on a hundred different tangents, ninety-nine of which may hurt the patient more than help him; but, if you can find it, there's almost always that one open road to success.

I also learned about prevention. I had always known that preventing was a much more vital function of psychiatry than curing—but now I realized that it was truly feasible. This was brought home to me rather dramatically during one of the forum meetings. One of the big shots in the area of prevention spoke to the group; an incident he cited concerned a riot in the Roxbury section of Boston where I grew up. The speaker was so pompous and so holier-than-thou that I couldn't begin to communicate with him, but it was very obvious to me that he didn't know a damn thing about conditions in Roxbury. Nevertheless, he was the psychiatric consultant to the school system and when the potential for violence arose, naturally everyone called him to find out what to do. At first he refused to do anything. Finally the pressure got so heavy he condescended at least to talk with the youths involved. He met with the militant Negro leadership and, through the mayor's office, succeeded in working out a compromise that stayed the violence temporarily.

He told us that being an arbitrator really wasn't his role, that he had stepped out of his role as a psychiatrist when he became an arbitrator. Well, Christ! what was the role? If being a psychiatrist doesn't include dealing with emotions when they get out of control, what does it include? If a psychiatrist can't step in and protect the public when violence threatens, then what can he do? Of course it was his role to prevent the potentially destructive riot from taking place. The psychiatrist must be concerned with preventing psychiatric disturbances and pathological emotional eruptions if he's going to be concerned about mental health at all. In other words, promoting mental health should be more a function of the psychiatrist than coping with mental illness.

I was at long last beginning to get somewhere in my quest for competency. I could see the psychiatric specialty for what it was—as opposed to what it should be. I could judge others in the field on the basis of their ability and not their pseudoauthority. I could confront guys like the big shot Boston consultant on any level because I realized that their powers were only transitory after all. They were actually the weak links in the field because they really didn't know a damn thing about psychiatry. Most significant, I had recognized the primary goals of psychiatry for what they were and was working toward them. I could now meet patients with confidence, assess their situations, and get to the foundation of their problems without fumbling all over the place for logical answers. I had found most of the answers I had been seeking.

When I knew I had accomplished what I had set out to do and felt myself falling into a rut, I left the Milwaukee clinic and went back into private practice. This time I was convinced of my ability; this time I was satisfied to call myself a psychiatrist, a competent psychiatrist. It had taken a grand total of twenty-two years. Tucson, Arizona would give me the room I needed in which to spread my newfound wings. I felt suffocated by the physical and human stench of the big cities. The time had come to breathe some fresh air, if that was possible.

IN THE FIELD

When I first saw J.B. a few years ago, he was in an extreme state of agitation. "You're the fifth psychiatrist I've been to in six months," he told me, "and if anything, I'm getting worse not better."

"Tell me about it," I suggested.

"Well, the first doctor told me it would take three to five years of daily sessions. At fifty bucks an hour, I couldn't afford it nor could I take all that time off from work. He thought I was just resisting, but that's ridiculous. The second doctor just gave me some pills and told me to cheer up, things would get brighter. The third guy gave me shock treatments, which helped for awhile, but then I began getting more depressed than ever. And that last one! He was a bigger nut than I am! I mean it! He had this thing about fresh air. Even though it was snowing, he had to have all the windows in the place open. I nearly froze to death before I got out of there. What's wrong with psychiatry anyway? Isn't there anybody around who knows how to make it work?"

I could only commiserate with this distraught man who, unknowingly, was echoing the cries of so many other confused patients I had seen through the years. Right now—today, the field of psychiatry is so ravaged by problems, three levels of problems—clinical and practical as well as theoretical—that naturally its practitioners are being tossed and torn by the storm. I'm not saying all psychiatrists are equally concerned with all problems in the field. The kid fresh out of training is going to be more bothered by the intellectual confusion than the guy out in the boondocks who is disgusted with the poor literature, or the crusader in the urban renewal area who spends more time arguing with city officials than he does in his treatment room. All three guys, in reality all psychiatrists, no matter what their ages, their training, their backgrounds, their speciaties, must grapple continuously with that one overwhelming quandry: the fact that psychiatry as a profession has not been channeled into a systematized body of knowledge and approach to problems (as has internal medicine, surgery, radiology, or any of the other branches of medicine).

You can well imagine what such a dilemma is doing to the practice of psychiatry. Since psychiatrists have medical degrees, they are expected to diagnose and treat patients with the competency and efficiency of other medical doctors, to be scientists in other words. Yet, the understanding of their specialty, human behavior, is not so much a science as it is an art; and to practice successful psychotherapy, psychiatrists must rely as much on intuition as on fact. Their medical orientation, therefore, confuses as much as it contributes to their psychotherapeutic function. After long years of medical training, all that the young psychiatrist actually has to put in his little black bag of nostrums is a conglomeration of ideas picked up during his residency along with a limited amount of practical experience, where he learned on a very empirical and pragmatic basis that sometimes certain things work and sometimes they don't. What he then has to do is organize an approach that he thinks will work with most patients. He tends to do this unconsciously rather than consciously and what he comes up with reflects his own personality more than it does the influence of his training or the impact of professional standards. Before he can make any attempt at effective psychotherapy, he has to develop some kind of methodological defense against the fact that there is no established method.

A few young shrinks have the guts to look the problem square in the face, to recognize it for the dilemma it is and place it in proper perspective. They are able to compromise theoretical formulations with clinical practice in a way that best benefits themselves, their patients, and their profession. It might take them years to master their weaknesses and perfect their expertise, to develop their artistry and expand their intellects. But once they have gone through the whole elusive hell of challenging mental illness and searching out the truths about it, once they have plummeted to the depths of despair and delusion and found their own individual, consistent, practical answers to it, they have earned the right to consider themselves healers of the mind. They have achieved the ultimate goal of true competency.

Most young psychiatrists, however, don't ever get this far. In their utter confusion they flutter all over the place trying to create an image for themselves somewhere between a doctor with a palette and an artist with a thermometer. It's a tremendous period of instability and disillusionment for them and they grab onto any likely pattern of adaptibility, usually one coinciding with one of the current problems in the field, that will help them pull themselves together enough to meet the public. With no professional design imposed upon them, with only their own inner voices telling them what to do and how to do it, these immature shrinks can and do go off in almost any direction. In other words, the kinds of psychiatrists they become is the result of their struggle with what the field has become and their own personal hang-ups. Their motives for choosing this line of work also play a significant role. Following are a few descriptions of the more abundant if less salient types that I have run across during my fifteen years in psychiatric practice.

THE IMITATION ANALYST

As far as these boys are concerned, there are no theoretical problems in psychiatry because there are no acceptable theories except psychoanalysis. To compensate for their own lack of identity, they latch onto Freud as the father figure of all time, revering his utterances, particularly the discussions of sexuality that somehow satisfy their own sexual frustrations and curiosities, as the very morsels of the divine. Unfortunately, they hear only the utterances they want to hear. They cling desperately to them long after they have been disproved, long after even Freud himself and other proponents of psychoanalysis have cast them aside. Dear old Ziggy changed his mind so many times during his creative years that even Anna had trouble keeping up with him, but the Imitator never changes his mind. He just hangs in there with his preconceived notions of human behavior and looks for things in patients that fit his theories rather than adapting his theories to the patient's symptoms.

The Imitator is not content with superficial understanding. He must work at "the deepest levels" of the mind, usually the level of infantile patterns of sexual and aggressive impulses, and make "dynamically oriented interpretations" of what his patients tell him. When a patient appears excessively jealous of her husband, for example, this must be traced to an incestuous wish for her father rather than, as is frequently the case, to the fact that hubby may be having an affair with his secretary. Like Freud, this type may sport a long beard, a beady-eyed expression and a condescending smirk. He seldom smiles, except at jokes no one else seems to understand.

There are competent psychoanalysts in the field, but watch out for the Imitator. Fantasy is more potent than reality to this shrink, and he might act out his fantasies at any time at the expense of the patient's real illness.

The idea that psychoanalytic theory is the one and only explanation of human behavior is the biggest fantasy of them all, but since this guy has gotten rid of his problems by believing it, he is convinced that he can lick his patient's problems with the same method.

THE DOKTOR

This species has never gotten over all that time spent in medical school and insists on playing the authoritarian doctor role despite the psychiatric consequences. These shrinks are convinced that psychiatry can be reduced to an applied science, like the other fields of medicine, and rather promiscuously dispense advice, write prescriptions, and turn on the shock box. They continue to use even the most primitive forms of organic therapy long after they have lost favor with other practicing psychiatrists and until society itself finally disapproves and turns thumbs down, e.g., insulin coma and lobotomy.

The layman is at a complete disadvantage with this licensed, white-coated, masterful figure who throws big words and psychiatric terms around with such erudite confidence and absolute ignorance. Though he appears benevolent because of the interest he takes in patients, he can, in fact, be very dangerous to those unaware that psychiatric diagnoses don't have the same meaning as medical diagnoses. A medical diagnosis is based on organic dysfunction requiring specific medical treatment and implies a general understanding of the illness by all doctors. If a patient has diabetes, his pancreas is not functioning properly and he requires insulin. A psychiatric diagnosis of this kind is meaningless. Psychiatric labels are much broader in scope and tell very little about individual pathology. Saying that a patient is schizophrenic reveals nothing about his specific symptoms, the causes of his illness or his prognosis; it merely indicates that at one time or other he was psychotic. Furthermore, psychiatrists are as apt to disagree on a diagnosis as they are to agree. Just as the Imitator believes in his theories, the Doktor has faith in his diagnoses and medications, as if Thorazine was an antischizophrenic drug the way insulin is an antidiabetic drug. Both approaches are high-handed, pseudo attempts to brainwash people into getting better without benefit of the kind of dialogue that must take place if real improvement is to occur. The Doktor type prefers to discuss patient symptoms in terms of how well they respond to prescribed medication rather than in terms of the underlying conflicts that perpetuate them. A flagrant example of this type was known endearingly in the community as "Electric Larry." When he wasn't pushing the button on the shock machine, he was handing out thyroid tablets for what he mistakenly considered to be subclinical cases of hypothyroidism.

For patients neurotically searching for a traditional doctor-patient relationship, this type would be glad to oblige, meanwhile reinforcing the pathology rather than relieving it. For patients with certain rigid religious backgrounds, organic therapy may be the most acceptable form of treatment. Sectarian hospitals are overrun with Doktor-type psychiatrists. For patients seeking permanent relief from their symptoms, a physiological approach is at best a stopgap and very frequently a complete waste of time and money.

THE PIGEON-HOLER

This guy copes with the theoretical bombardment by becoming neutral, by keeping himself at arm's length from any problem and any way to solve it. He's a cousin to the Doktor type as he likes to pin labels on patients, but he's a step ahead of the Doktor in realizing that he doesn't know very much, even about medicine. He also has some of the Imitator's characteristics, some of the less positive ones, but doesn't allow himself to become so involved in dyamics.

The Pigeon-Holer approaches all patients and all patient problems objectively, so objectively that he never gets emotionally entangled or shares any of the patient's real anxieties. He has almost a compulsion to reduce all symptoms to simplistic, judgmental value terms, to sort them out according to some precise little mental file of his own derivation. Once categorized, a patient is there to stay. The Pigeon-Holer is much too rigid to shift labels and much too empty and shallow to respond or relate to anyone on a human, one-to-one level, including even his own family. He is not really a psychiatrist or a human being. He is merely a good actor playing the roles of both.

Pigeon-Holers are always gentlemen. Since they never get their hands dirty or their emotions aroused, they have no reason to be otherwise. Waspy, distinguished looking citizens, they are highly respected in the community and well liked in their neighborhoods because they invariably do and say the right things. They cater to the prevailing fads of the community, serving those committees they think the psychiatrist is supposed to become involved with in order to maintain the image. Little or nothing is ever really accomplished. They are particularly active in the legal system, for courts require black and white answers to questions of human behavior, and these birds are able to give them in good conscience. They are also comfortable in the role of consultants to other social agencies because they reduce problems to such simplistic terms, they virtually eliminate them. The Pigeon-Holer has his own life and conflicts in order at all times and proudly maintains complete control over the few emotions that manage to slip through. That's the performance he thinks a psychiatrist should give. But it isn't even human.

THE SWINGER

This is a new breed of psychiatrist. Largely disillusioned with traditional forms of psychotherapy, he latches on to any new approach he happens to read about in the journals or hear about at the meetings he attends. Today he may be turned on by gestalt therapy and encounter groups; tomorrow it may be reality therapy or psychodrama. His enthusiasms run the gamut from behavioral modification (where all human behavior is put on a basis of punishment and reward) to crisis intervention (treating the wound before it has time to fester) to group therapy (or letting patients treat each other) to you name it.

When you place yourself in the hands of the Swinger, you're resorting to psychiatric roulette. This guy plays games with his patients hoping to find one that will make them better, and there aren't any rules to his games. He, too, likes role playing to a certain extent, acting out the patient's problems to further intensify the conflict situations. Or maybe he'll find it more fun to manipulate the patient's environment than to try to win the real hassle with the conflicts. If he gets desperate he'll even go to extremes. In at least one case, a Swinger told a depressed patient to go out and have an affair with somebody new, that her problems came from boredom with her old mate. Needless to say, this advice did not make him very popular with the patient's husband.

The Swinger tends to be younger than the other types and has a flair for making a good first impression. If involved primarily in community psychiatry, he's always making the local headlines for setting up new programs for mentally ill, frequently usurping the credit of less glory-seeking, more unobtrusive workers. He gets quoted for making profound statements such as "marijuana may have some use in the treatment of depression" or "this patient needs to figure out what she herself wants" when the patient is semicatatonic and unable to figure out anything. This guy may come on strong but rapidly fizzles out when people realize that he frequently doesn't know what he's talking about, and his latest fad is exposed as the superficial type of quackery it really is. Like the camera of the same name, our Swinger is quick to espouse a new form but slow to control its quality.

THE ORGANIZATION MAN

This character doesn't even try to think for himself but gets his direction from an organization, be it mental hospital, medical school department of psychiatry, state department of mental health, or national professional association. He seeks political and professional status by heading up this and directing that, somehow feeling that by becoming a big wheel in psychiatry, he will in some magical way be transformed into a competent psychiatrist like the big shot consultant I mentioned earlier. He mistakenly equates power with performance. Having achieved these positions largely by virtue of the "Peter principle" (in any organization a person rises to his level of incompetence), he is characteristically a poor administrator and the only real power he has is in making life miserable for those under him. Competent people in his employ don't take him too seriously until he finally botches things up so badly they can't afford to ignore him.

The Organizer doesn't like working with patients and takes advantage of organized ways to get rid of them—therapy groups, hospitals, or supervised recreational sessions. He forms no relationships with patients; he keeps them dangling at arm's length. Since he is more often than not a social misfit and unable to relate to normal people, it isn't surprising that he can form no

bond with the mentally ill. Nor does he become personally or professionally involved in their problems but
relies on his organizational network to probe into them
or plan them away. In the community, this guy's bag is
politics and public clinics. He does wield a kind of
negative power here since he's the one who usually
determines what kind of research will be funded and
who will get the grants. Since political considerations
on his part will better enhance his position, he is more
inclined to make decisions that are expedient for him
rather than essential for the field.

Organizational structures in the mental health field
today are so tenuous that it is rare for any chief of psychiatry to last very long. This is, perhaps, one of the few
advantages of the current chaotic American scene. Beware of the chief. He needs Indians to support his narcis-
sism, but patients don't need a chief. They need a proper
sounding board to elicit their underlying conflicts and
help redirect their energies along more constructive
lines.

THE PROBLEM SHRINK

Since all psychiatrists are human, all psychiatrists have problems of one sort or another. However, I
would guess that about one in six have problems so severe
that they are sicker than most of their patients. I have
known shrinks who were alcoholic, drug addicted, homosexual, neurotic, psychotic, and combinations of all of
these. They are social misfits in the truest sense and are
definitely problems to themselves and almost everyone
with whom they associate.

These are the boys who went into psychiatry looking
for answers for themselves rather than for patients.
Their problems can vary in intensity and form—one guy
I know gets so scared when he meets new people that

he shakes like a victim of St. Vitus' Dance—but their presence on any level unqualifiedly complicates any attempt at psychotherapy. J.B.'s fifth shrink is a perfect example. In addition, these poor creatures are so insecure and dependent themselves, they promote this kind of regression in their patients. They go overboard in becoming involved with patients, overidentifying with them, projecting their own warped personalities onto them, even going so far as suggesting the personal crutches and panaceas that they themselves find beneficial. It would not be at all unusual for the Problem Psychiatrist to ask a depressed patient, "Have you ever gotten drunk? I used to find a few drinks very helpful for depression." Or a frigid female, "Have you tried an affair with a guy who really knows his anatomy? If you'll let me, I think I could get you over this hang-up once and for all." Problem Shrinks think nothing of discussing their own problems with the patient, and in some instances it becomes a question of just who's treating whom.

Psychiatrists with problems tend to rely too heavily on sedatives and potentially addictive medications, both for themselves and their patients. They sustain all concerned indefinitely in a nether world of artificial stimulation and relaxation without ever getting down to the basis of the real problems involved. But patients keep coming back to be sustained. Why shouldn't they? It gives them a feeling of well-being to see someone sicker than themselves and besides, the Problem Shrink is so good to them, giving them anything and everything they supposedly need and want. Patients may come away loving this jerk, never realizing how destructive he actually is.

THE GOOD JOE

He solves everything with love. He's really unbalanced because one eye is blind and the other responds too well. In the business of love versus hate, he overresponds to love and ignores hate because his own emotional need for approval allows him to see only half the picture. He is completely incapable of coping with his own hostilities and aggressions, much less anybody else's so his technique is to dote on patients, never asserting himself, never taking a firm stand on anything, just placating away day after day, year after year. He has tremendous difficulty terminating the therapy, all in the name of concern for the patient, like an overprotective mother. The Good Joe is a big breast to his patients, as if by feeding them enough of the milk of human kindness their hostilities will just float away.

Good Joes also like to spread love around the community. They have a way of monopolizing community affairs and are all over the place "doing good," not only on an individual but on a group level as well. They're going to solve the whole community's problems, and, of course, the only thing they ever accomplish is to become hopelessly enmeshed in never-ending discussions that usually lead nowhere and are seldom of real value. But they go on discussing anyway because they're so great at pussyfooting around and uttering mealy-mouthed platitudes of one sort or another that the naïve public thinks, "Oh, isn't that smart! Isn't that marvelous!" Religion is one of Good Joe's favorite topics, and he frequently forms associations with the clergy. These aren't productive either because good old insipid Joe is so fearful of offending his clerical buddies that he steers clear of the issues that should be talked about—areas of conflict between the two fields.

Sadly enough, this type probably has a pretty good grasp of basic dynamics. He might even acquire an adequate understanding of the patient's conflicts. His desire to please is greater than his desire to confront the patient with those things he has to be confronted with in order to get well. Intellectually, Good Joe recognizes the patient's needs but emotionally he just can't bring it off. It frightens me when I see how many of these jokers are out there trying to practice psychotherapy. If only they could shit or get off the pot, perhaps they could become useful with some patients anyway!

THE COMPETENT PSYCHIATRIST

At the end of his twelve years of medical education, a guy comes out thinking he's a big shot headshrinker. He knows what makes you tick and how to help you, you poor bastards who are neurotic and psychotic and terribly depressed. And, of course, he doesn't. His training, all twelve years of it, has been too meager, his instruction too discombobulated, his clinical work too limited. His real training starts now, but very few freshly graduated young shrinks have the right combination of internal ingredients—the perseverance, the curiosity, the elasticity, or the maturity—to come to grips with the many problems in the field of psychiatry and with their own inability to cope with them. They need to keep their egos in perspective and not rationalize their weaknesses into false strengths, to work diligently and constantly at their own lives, keeping themselves adaptable and in good mental health. Those who do, eventually become competent psychiatrists.

Of course, they pay a big price for it. They go through hell, as I did, struggling with all types of problems—theoretical, practical, administrative, personal, and unresolvable. Then there are the doubts, the frustrations, the hurts, the questions, the errors, and finally some of the successes. They pay in blood and sweat and tears, in sleepless nights, in tired bodies, and in confused minds. They pay for a number of years after they have completed their residencies, and at no time do they fall back on any of the phony mechanisms for dealing with difficult situations. They learn to recognize problems and then find ways to deal with them. They learn to be comfortable within themselves, to depend on their own emotional stability, to have confidence so that they can relate to patients on two levels subtly and simultaneously: the personal and the professional. They learn to be much more flexible than their initial training ever taught them to be, to reconcile apparently conflicting schools of thought, to develop therapeutic relationships with all kinds of people from all kinds of backgrounds. They learn all of this basically, through relating to patients, maybe never dealing with the problems directly or verbally, but always being aware of them and working them out in the best way they know how.

A Competent Psychiatrist neither seeks nor attracts a great deal of publicity or community recognition. Yet other physicians are well aware of him because most of the patients they refer to him improve. His greatest attribute is his ability to adapt his techniques to the specific needs of his patients, but without confusing directness of approach for misguided flexibility. He gives firm direction to characterologically disturbed patients. He guides depressed patients in the catharsis of ambivalent feelings toward the lost loved one. He helps neurotics to uncover the reasons for their neurosis. He escorts psychotics back to reality while minimizing the shame involved. He only becomes involved with other social agencies when the welfare of his patients demands it—and then he does so quite vigorously.

The Competent Psychiatrist does not hide behind technical jargon or medical authority. He has no single theoretical bias but borrows from all theories as the needs of his patients dictate. He does not squeak when he should roar, does not avoid meeting patients head on and confronting them with their problems. Neither does he jump out and frighten patients assaulting them with revelations before they are ready and adding to their already existing traumas. Being primarily a clinician, the Competent Psychiatrist does not want to be bogged down by administrative hassles and, therefore, is seldom motivated to become a chief of psychiatry or a chairman of a department. I don't know how many of these men are in practice today, certainly not many, definitely not enough, probably too few to make themselves heard against the din of inadequacies causing the current crisis. Those who are around have a big job ahead if they're going to make effective inroads into the more defeating problems, if they're going to lead the field by example to more productivity and more accomplishment.

I have presented these personality profiles not to explode the myth of the psychiatrist but to expose him in all his human idiosyncrasies—a human being who may or may not be qualified to treat mental illness. As I have colored them, my "types" appear to be pretty clearly delineated, but undoubtedly there are few, if any, actual therapists who fit these pictures exactly. More accurately, individuals tend to develop into a combination of types such that one might be 75 percent the Doktor and 25 percent the Problem, another might be 90 percent Good Joe and 10 percent Competent. That's an important point, that business of being occasionally competent, because it's all too true that some psychiatrists can deal adequately with certain problems even though they may be worse than adequate with others. Although Good Joes can't tolerate aggression, for instance, some of them handle frustrated females quite well. It all depends on the guy himself, what his inner resources are, what his background has been, how he has come to terms with that big question in psychiatry—art versus science.

A psychiatrist is no better than his capacity to understand and treat patients. The better psychiatrists have the higher batting averages. They help more people because they have more talent and are better at their jobs. As with any other true professional, a psychiatrist's reward is not the twenty-five or fifty bucks an hour, it is the intuitive awareness of a job well done. In our materialistic society, it is little wonder that competent psychotherapy is so hard to come by, that lousy psychotherapy abounds everywhere, and that all gradations in between are thriving. Because psychiatry is just like anything else in modern life, you pay your money and you get taken, unless you stand up for your rights and demand competency.

IN ACTION

Most patients I see are overly concerned about schools of psychiatry, when they should be thinking about the personal style of the psychiatrist. They come into my office wanting to know if I'm Freudian, Frommian, Sullivanian, or what the hell I am. All psychiatrists, even those claiming to be eclectic, have some point of view and certainly the patient is entitled to know what direction his headshrinker leans toward. Practically speaking, however, the schools of psychiatry are not well defined. Since there is no totally comprehensive theory of human behavior, there is no one school of psychiatry that has all the answers. Therefore, no shrink who adheres rigidly to any one dictate is going to be able to treat all varieties of human disturbance.

The practice of psychiatry is more related to the brand of therapy practiced than to a particular school. As I have already pointed out, psychiatrists are much more identifiable by their personal approaches to problems than by the particular precepts they preach. So how meaningful is it, really, when a shrink says, "I believe in the existential approach," or "I believe in the Adlerian approach"? Is he talking about the universal concerns of life and death? Is he talking about the struggle for emotional survival and how to make the most of it while you're going through it? Or is he just all wrapped up in some masturbatory fantasy that he had last night— coping with one small wound while the very mortality gushes out of the patient?

After spending more than six months in psychotherapy with five different shrinks J.B., too, began to realize that there might be many possible approaches to a problem but only one or two proper ones. His history was pretty typical. J.B. is a thirty-one-year-old single executive in a plastics firm. He has been with the company only five years but because of his drive and affable nature is being groomed for a top management position. J.B. was in love with a beautiful and talented young lady. Just when he was considering marriage, he began to suffer increasing symptoms of anxiety, depression, and inability to make a final commitment to her. The prospect of marriage panicked him. He avoided her for increasingly long intervals. He spent his time playing tennis or on the golf course or just having a few drinks with the boys. He had recently met and was having an affair with a woman who was somewhat younger than his fiancée and couldn't make up his mind between them. J.B. was working as hard as ever on the job, and his symptoms did not impair his efficiency there. It was only when he allowed himself to dwell on the problem that he would break out in a cold sweat and have palpitations. He was becoming sexually impotent with his fiancée. The idea of marriage to her was associated in his mind with the fear that it would lead eventually to a very boring kind of stalemate and after a few years probably end in divorce.

J.B. was obviously of above average intelligence, handsome and rugged in personal appearance. He was quite athletic and competitive. At a relatively tender age, he had decided that he was going to be successful not only in sports but in the business world as well. This was in marked contrast to his father who had tried a number of business enterprises, all of which had ended in failure. As a child he could recall that when his mother made disparaging remarks about his father, he would be considerably upset though he generally tended to agree with her. Though he loved his father personally, he tended to despise him as a man. J.B. had a number of problems, none of them too serious in their present stage, but all of them potentially dangerous if allowed to go untreated. In the face of this inadequate therapy, J.B. himself had noted that his symptoms were getting progressively worse. We now examine how each type of psychiatrist would handle his case, further illustrating the various techniques of psychotherapy being practiced today.

The Imitation Analyst, as previously illustrated, would tend to discourage him on the basis of the amount of time and money that the treatment would envolve. He would probably focus on the patient's castration anxiety. J.B.'s depression would be analyzed in terms of a fear of following in his father's footsteps and the resultant inability to live up to the self-image he had created of an extremely virile male who could admit to no weakness or shortcoming. Eventually, he would focus on latent homosexuality as an explanation for why J.B. preferred to go drinking with the boys rather than to settle down to marriage with his fiancee. He would then go on to an analysis of the patient's dreams, hoping to find an incestuous tie between J.B. and his mother. As a final coup, he would encourage J.B. to form a neurotic negative transference to him that would take years to analyze away before he would pronounce the patient cured.

The Doktor would immediately check J.B.'s past medical history for any illness, such as mumps orchitis, that might affect sexual potency. He would tend to be supporting in a general way—"Of course, it's difficult for you to make a decision about marriage, and naturally you would tend to have a certain amount of conflict about this"—never finding out why this decision was so uniquely difficult for him. If his superficial techniques of reassurance and pills didn't work, he would call on his heavier artillery—increased drug dosages, possible shock treatments, knocking the patient into oblivion until he forgot about the underlying causes of his symptoms the way the Doktor himself had.

The Pigeon-Holer would immediately categorize him as a sexually inadequate male who compensated for this by his excessive devotion to work and duty. He would say that J.B.'s symptoms had developed simply because this basic sexual inadequacy had caught up with him when he was under the pressure of finally having to make a decision to get married. He would tend conveniently to overlook the fact that J.B.'s sexual adjustment had been quite satisfactory up to the point where the possibility of marriage had entered the picture. He would simply prescribe a mild tranquilizer and suggest that he get even more involved in his work and sports activities. He would not see the patient very often and would develop no real relationship with him. Furthermore, if J.B. didn't show rapid signs of improvement, he would become uncomfortable with him. Knowing that his therapist was rejecting him and loathing the person he had categorized him as being, J.B. would end up playing the role, kidding himself into thinking he was better just to get rid of the Pigeon-holer. In a short time he would be knocking at someone else's door.

By definition it is hard to predict what direction the Swinger would take. He might relate to J.B. by focusing on his sexual adjustment to the new girlfriend. Even though the patient had told him that his sexual adjustment with his fiancée had been satisfactory previously, the Swinger might keep looking for something wrong in this area. He might get the fiancée in on the act and treat them both in his so-called couple's therapy, thus diluting J.B.'s individual treatment. He might try a bit of psychodrama. He could take the role of the fiancée himself and ask J.B. what he would say to her, perhaps getting him so stirred up that in the end he might become even more depressed and possibly suicidal.

The Organizer might put J.B. on some antianxiety medication right away and suggest that he go ahead and live with his fiancée for awhile on a kind of trial basis. If this bit of environmental manipulation did not work and the symptoms worsened, he would be quick to hospitalize him, throwing him into a routine of milieu therapy and giving little consideration to J.B.'s real psychological needs. Whether an inpatient or an outpatient, he would schedule him for group therapy although he couldn't define it, explain how it works, or tell what patients are best suited for it. Some anxious male patients of this type become more agitated when they hear about other people's problems, but it goes against the Organizer's grain to make exceptions.

The Problem Shrink will prescribe sedatives, stimulants, and any other drugs that J.B. requests. He will become very friendly with him on a personal basis, telling him all about his own past experiences and the difficulties he has had with women. He might well bring up his own marital situation and regale the patient with the vicissitudes of that relationship and how he coped with them. If he uses drugs, he will encourage him to use drugs. If he drinks, he will suggest alcohol. If he takes bare-footed walks in the rain, he will have J.B. out wading during the monsoons. He will see him frequently, and their relationship will travel from the office to long friend-ly chats in the neighborhood bar. He will never get around to J.B.'s basic problems and the best ways of deal-ing with them.

Good Joe will probably tell him that he is overly concerned about the future of the marriage. That his lack of confidence is based simply on his father's prev-ious difficulties saying, "You've got to be strong and not allow the uncertainties of the future to get the better of you." After all, he doesn't want to arouse J.B.'s animosity. Since he perceives J.B. as actually a more successful male than he is himself, he cannot deal with the dynamics of J.B.'s neurotic conflict. To do so would mean to mobil-ize all of the negative feelings J.B. unconsciously har-bors toward the important people in his life. Good Joe is afraid these hostile feelings will be transferred onto him. Consequently, he will gloss over the underlying problems hoping that all the love and good will he is offering will be enough to get J.B. well. He will keep him in therapy indefinitely, giving him lots of advice for handling every-day problems and fostering his increasing dependence on him. The day of reckoning will come, however, and J.B.'s fruitless search for a competent psychiatrist may soon end in complete desperation.

Though there may be a grain of truth in all these approaches, none is really on target. The Competent Psychiatrist might borrow from some of them but regard-less of the method he chooses, he will go right to the heart of the matter, namely, J.B.'s fear of commiting himself to one particular woman. While maintaining a positive professional relationship with him, being sympathetic but not overly so, he will encourage him to expose any unresolved conflicts he has with his fiancée and to call forth all of the memories and associations related to this fear from his earlier life. He will explore in depth J.B.'s relationship with his fiancée as well as the meaning of his turning to the second girl. He will analyze the meaning of J.B.'s tremendous drive to achieve and help him gradually to understand the reasons for it in terms of his relationship both with his father and mother. That he perceives women as being constantly detrimental to the successful pursuit of a career will also be fully dealt with in the treatment. The Competent Psychiatrist does not judge his patient; he treats him. He does not encourage dependency; rather, he helps his patient to become first interdependent with and then independent of him. If he needs a mild tranquilizer or an antidepressant he will prescribe it. He does not experiment on him with half-baked theories or untested hypotheses. He hears his problems and helps him solve them for himself.

With this kind of intelligent, intensive, individual therapy, patients such as J.B. are able to get well in a short time. As a matter of fact, with once-a-week sessions over a six-month period, J.B. did respond very well and went on to build a rich and rewarding life, grateful that he had finally gotten the help he needed. I saw him once following his marriage and all of the old anxieties had disappeared. He was less compulsively driven in terms of his job performance, but still doing an excellent job. I filed J.B.'s folder among the inactive cases and found myself wishing they could all be so easy. Why don't more psychiatrists deal with the real psychological problems of their patients rather than just compulsively repeating their own methodological defenses against the ambiguities that exist in the field of psychiatry? The real psychiatrist will stand up, but you have to ask him first to do so.

CHAPTER **3**

Will The Real Patient
Please Stand Up

OVER THE YEARS, I have seen people in consultation who did not really need a psychiatrist. I have seen
some who needed one but were unable to accept the fact.
A few have been able to accept the fact and yet were
unable to go through with the therapy. Others have come
to find out whether or not they could benefit from psychiatric treatment. After discussing their problems briefly,
they will confront me on their first visit with, "Do I need
a headshrinker or don't I?" I find this approach refreshing because it generally means that the person in question is open minded and flexible, and will respond
constructively.

Everyone has occasional trouble making decisions.
This does not mean we all need help. Most people develop
psychosomatic symptoms at one time or another, and
they don't require psychotherapy. Under conditions of
severe stress, many people have wondered if it wouldn't
be easier just to end it all, but that isn't always an

indication for treatment either. All people experience anxiety or depression periodically; they don't all have to dash for the nearest mental health center. You need a psychiatrist when you are hurting so badly that you begin to feel there is no solution to your problem. That is the very critical psychological threshold beyond which you should not push yourself. To do so would only complicate matters further.

Take the guy who is contemplating suicide. Like anyone else, he may just be wondering what it would be like to be dead. He may even get a certain thrill out of reflecting briefly on the various methods of taking his own life. The basic difference between this guy's relatively normal mental masturbation and true psychiatric disturbance is the degree of intensity. When a patient thinks about killing himself, he becomes extremely tense and fearful lest he lose control and blow his brains out or jump off the nearest skyscraper. It's not just an idle thought that passes through his mind; it's something he dwells on at length and becomes really up tight about. The same thing occurs with other symptoms. Depression lingers and becomes difficult to shake off. Psychosomatic symptoms persist and intensify. Anxiety becomes chronic when the initial crisis has long since passed.

Everyone knows that acutely psychotic patients need psychiatric help as quickly as possible. Acute psychosis, however, accounts for only a small percentage of the mental illness in this country. The vast majority suffer from far less dramatic manifestations, some of them so mild that it may be difficult to decide whether a psychiatrist is or is not necessary. Since admittedly we all have our troubles, our individual quirks, how is it possible for the layman to tell when certain situations are beyond rationalizing as the "fast pace of modern life" or so and so's "little eccentricities"? Are there any reliable criteria for making this kind of judgment?

SIX REASONS TO STAND UP

Psychiatric problems usually present themselves in one of six ways:
1. a stressful life situation or personal crisis,
2. a psychosomatic symptom including anxiety and depression along with any other type of physical complaint,
3. a prepsychotic state of mind,
4. a full-blown psychosis, or
5. a behavior disorder or a problem that the friends or relatives must cope with.

LIFE SITUATION OR PERSONAL CRISIS

Probably the simplest category, at least from the psychiatric viewpoint, is the life problem. A person comes up against a situation in his everyday life that he just doesn't know how to handle; frequently, he has to make some sort of decision but is unsure of himself. He has reached an impasse, feeling that he's damned if he does and damned if he does not. He tries to solve the problem but things only get worse. He talks to friends, to people at the office, to neighbors, to his family doctor, and anyone else who will listen. He still can't make any headway. He is preoccupied with the situation, becoming restless at night and, therefore, less efficient by day. Both his peace of mind and his capacity to relax are jeopardized. He can't shrug it off and he can't solve it.

When any life problem has reached these proportions, it is time to take it to a competent psychiatrist. He will help you deal with it far more effectively than you could alone, tracing it back to its origins, bringing the past into broader perspective with the present, and showing you why you have become so emotionally involved in the problem. Most life situations, which patients have struggled with for months, require only a few sessions with a competent psychiatrist. A typical response of such a patient after a few sessions is, "You know, I never quite thought of it that way. You're right; I don't know how I could have allowed myself to get so worked up when the answer was so obvious." When this happens, it means that the patient has achieved a certain amount of emotional insight, and he can then pick up the pieces and resume his life.

I treated a physician who, with no prior history of emotional disorder, was completely thrown by having to retire from a very active practice for physical reasons. He was sixty-five-years-old and had been a workhorse all his life. He had never cultivated any hobbies nor had he developed any real interests outside of his immediate family and his profession. He was simply unable to accept this mandatory retirement, feeling that he had nothing left to live for and regretting the fact that the heart attack hadn't actually killed him. He became seriously depressed and difficult to motivate, spending much of his time in obsessive thinking of the past, wishing that he had done certain things and regretting that he had done others.

His case is typical of older men facing forced retirement. Some of them learn to accept their physical limitations and work out their feelings on their own by engaging in part-time work, traveling, or spending more time with their families. Others, especially those of middle-class background and compulsive personality structure, tend to dwell on the fact that they, the breadwinners for so long, have suddenly become invalids. The more important their work was to them and the more constricted their outside interests, the tougher they will be to treat. Their self-respect was always equated with job performance and when the latter is taken away from, the former dries up and disappears. I never cease to be amazed by the fact that so many people in our society are completely unprepared for retirement. From the looks of things though, the younger generation is not about to let this happen to them. Many of them seem to be demanding that they be allowed to live lives of perpetual retirement. It's not strange, is it, that one extreme tends to breed its opposite?

A graduate student who had to complete his Ph.D. dissertation by a certain date became so up tight about it that he couldn't work on it. Although brilliant in his highly specialized field, he had a history of putting things off until the last minute. He could express himself quite well verbally, but when it came to writing a paper, he tended to freeze. He would not get his degree unless he completed his thesis successfully, and a failure to do so would prevent his achieving any kind of success in his chosen field. Though completing written assignments may cause any student a few headaches and may normally even lead to a few sleepless nights, for this student, it was a crisis situation. He needed psychiatric help because he was unable to settle down to the task at hand; had he not received the help, he might well have blown his whole future.

A life situation became a psychiatric problem in the case of a young woman who miscarried her first child at six months of pregnancy. When she came in, she was extremely despondent about the loss and harbored feelings of inadequacy for not having brought the baby live into the world. All women who lose babies do not become pathologically depressed. A certain amount of grief is normal. This woman, however, blamed herself for what had happened and required a few sessions in therapy before she could forgive and forget. She was then able to anticipate future pregnancies without fearing that the same thing would happen again.

A mandatory retirement, a deadline that has to be met, or a miscarriage that has to be accepted—these are the experiences of life that people frequently get hung up on to the point where psychiatric care is indicated. Indeed, any common life situation can develop into a major hassle: trying to decide whether to marry or divorce, how to discipline the children; finding ways to cope with a rebellious adolescent, an unwanted pregnancy, a mother who has a fatal illness; or anything that comes along to stir up problems that begin to get the better of the individual.

The most common cause of distress is the marital problem. I would guess that more than half the life problems I see are brought about by disturbed marriages. A disturbed marriage is any marriage in which one of the partners feels there is something wrong in the relationship. These marital problems usually turn out to be much more complicated than is generally recognized, either in the professional literature or in the lay publications. Couples generally wait too long before seeking help. Both usually have their own individual hang-ups as well as suffer from the pathological interaction between the two of them. It is difficult to pinpoint one specific problem since, at any given time, the focus may be on one partner or the other or the interplay between them. Getting both the husband and wife to agree to treatment is frequently a chore. The husband might well be the one who needs the most help but will refuse to come in. He wants to believe that he is lily white and it's all his wife's fault. The psychiatrist may then have to work primarily through the wife in order to try to save the marriage, assuming that she herself wants to do so. It is, then, frequently the person who experiences the need for help most acutely who seeks psychiatric attention, not the one who actually needs it most. Regardless of which partner discovers the problem, he should first discuss the need for psychiatric consultation with his spouse. If the latter does not consent —and it is not at all unusual for one of the partners to hold out for quite awhile before finally conceding that outside help is needed—it will be up to the psychiatrist in conjunction with the patient to decide how to break the deadlock.

After four years of marriage, one man told his wife that he wanted to have sexual relations with other women and wanted to participate in orgies. She told me of his insisting that she make dates with other men and then bring them home in order to participate in various sexual activities—sometimes she and the other man alone, sometimes with the husband included, and sometimes with other women as well. Not wanting to go along with him, she acquiesced because she was afraid she would lose him otherwise, but she was in a constant state of turmoil. The husband absolutely refused to come anywhere near my office. He didn't see anything wrong with his behavior and was enjoying himself far too much to have anyone point out to him that it was a source of intense conflict for his wife. Since he refused to come in, I could only work toward building up the wife's self-confidence so that the fear of losing her husband would not prevent her from asserting her own feelings in the situation—a compromise solution, to be sure, but the best that could be achieved under the circumstances. Like any other psychiatric problem, the longer a marital conflict goes untreated, the more difficult it is to resolve. With the increasing popularity of sexual freedom, people who cannot personally accept this kind of behavior are having tremendous difficulty when confronted by members of their own families who casually indulge in sexual freedom.

Even when both partners are willing to accept treatment, the psychiatrist may choose any number of ways of handling their specific case. Sometimes I see husband and wife separately; at other times I may bring them together for certain sessions. In other instances, I may restrict the treatment to just one of the parties involved. Every marriage has its own characteristics and each case has to be dealt with on its own merits. For this reason any marital conflict, whether brought about by sex, money, children, in-laws, job, or whatever, that is serious enough to merit professional intervention should be evaluated by a competent psychiatrist. Let him decide who should be seen and how often.

Thirty-nine is a popular age for bringing to a head marital conflicts that may have long lain dormant. One husband had been having transient affairs with women for years, but at the magic age of thirty-nine decided he had found true love at last, in the person of his young secretary. Feeling ashamed, he decided he had better tell his wife, not only about the secretary, but about the other women as well. The wife found his confession overwhelming despite the fact she had been suspicious in the past.

For years the husband had been driven by strong achievement goals, working long hours and traveling. The wife had contributed to their gradual estrangement by often participating in outside activities that occupied her day and night for months at a time. On a conscious level, this couple had always assumed that they had an ideal marriage and had taken their relationship for granted. Except for the fact of keeping these activities secret from his wife, the husband had not really felt guilty about the previous sexual escapades because there had been no genuine emotional involvement. He felt his actions were just par for the course for a successful young executive, part of the image.

The qualitative difference between the purely physical attraction for the other women and the more emotional bond toward the secretary stirred up conflicts within him. For a long time he had a "madonna-prostitute" complex in relation to his wife, that is, he was able to accept her in the role of wife and mother but not in her sexual role. At the same time, he recognized that his attraction to the secretary was extremely immature; the girl herself was twenty years younger and emotionally unstable, and they really had nothing in common outside the bedroom. This kind of triangular relationship might have continued indefinitely had the husband not suddenly decided to confess everything to his wife.

Actually, this couple needed a psychiatrist long before the crisis in their marriage finally drove them to one. There were three patients in this case—the wife, the husband, and the neurotic marital relationship. Depending on the circumstances from week to week, I saw either husband or wife and occasionally both together. Had these people recognized their need for psychiatry when the process of estrangement had its onset many years ago, their treatment would have been far simpler and their personal lives far less disrupted.

Marital counseling can be one of the most difficult forms of psychotherapy and certainly shouldn't be entrusted to amateurs. This does not mean that psychiatry can always repair a jagged relationship—far from it. Nor does a divorce indicate that the therapy has failed. When I take on a case of maritial counseling, I explain to both parties that I cannot predict the outcome. In the course of the treatment, I give them my impressions and indicate clearly the conditions that have to be met by each of them in order for the marriage to work. In the event that both parties cannot meet the conditions, divorce is sometimes the only alternative. The termination of a marriage may not be an ideal solution but, in actual practice, it may be the only feasible one.

The vast majority of people considering separation or divorce need psychiatric counseling. The least that a competent psychiatrist can do in such a case is help the person remove any lingering doubts and clarify the reasons for his decision. This in itself will help prevent the recurrence of a similar situation. So often people do not understand why their marriages have gone awry and will embark on a second, only to repeat the same mistakes. With appropriate help, such mistakes and all the misery that accompanies them can be avoided.

PSYCHOSOMATIC SYMPTOM

Like the person confronted by an intolerable life situation, the patient who suffers from a specific symptom, whether anxiety, depression, or a psychosomatic disorder, feels unable to cope with it. These specific symptoms usually have their onset during times of stress, but they outlive their usefulness. Whereas anxiety is normally a signal that the person must be on the alert to handle a specific situation, in these cases, the situation has long since passed, but the person's mind and body react as if it were still present. Many people will have butterflies before taking an examination or asking the boss for a raise. A fast pulse is not unusual when your plane is about to take off. When the symptoms won't go away, however, when the anxieties, fears, depression, fatigue, nausea, or palpitations are far out of proportion to the realities involved, it's time, then, to seek psychiatric aid.

Included in this category are the many types of phobia from which people suffer, such as a fear of germs or a fear of closed places or a fear of impending doom. One very common form of anxiety and fear is known as hyperventilation, during which a person experiences various symptoms including dizziness, chest pain, fatigue, and

numbness or tingling of the extremities. In cases of hyperventilation, the fear leads to overbreathing that, in turn,
upsets the body's chemistry and results in physical symptoms. Such patients are apt to fear for their lives, thinking they are going to die at any moment. They also are
afraid of leaving the house, of being alone, or of losing
their minds. The initial episode of hyperventilation is
usually related to a very traumatic episode, frequently
pertaining to the death of a loved one. In susceptible
people, however, it goes on to become a self-perpetuating
vicious cycle: the symptoms themselves lead to more
anxiety, and the anxiety leads to more hyperventilation,
etc.

Most psychosomatic illnesses are handled very
poorly by the majority of physicians in this country. Too
many doctors merely brush them aside as insignificant
because they are unable to pinpoint any specific organic
basis for the symptoms. The notorious lack of finesse
that some doctors demonstrate in handling patients
psychologically has in fact created many psychiatric
problems.

The term "psychosomatic" has even become a dirty
word in many circles. To many people it means that the
symptoms are imaginary or unreal. Nothing could be further from the truth. The aches and pains are not manufactured by the patient merely to attract attention and
get a lot of sympathy from other people. These symptoms invariably reflect a state of chronic emotional
tension that simply can't find any other outlet! Patients
with such symptoms have learned at an early age to
repress all of their basic human emotions. To express
any kind of ordinary human frailty is equated with a state
of weakness and inferiority. Consequently, their emotional tensions seek a physiological outlet. Fearful of losing
control and afraid that other people will laugh at them if

they express their feelings directly, they have learned over the years to always appear strong in the eyes of other people. This defense mechanism gradually weakens, and then the body takes over and does its own thing. Any organ system of the body may be involved: respiratory, gastrointestinal, central nervous system, skin, genital, urinary, or any other.

Take a thirty-seven-year-old laborer who had burning of the penis for at least six months before I first saw him. As do most patients with psychosomatic illnesses, he denied, in the initial interview, having any emotional problems. He was completely preoccupied with the constant, painful sensation of burning throughout his genital organ, and he was certain that some physical disease was effecting it. Despite several medical examinations, including one by a urologist, all of which were entirely negative, he was convinced that the doctors had overlooked the basic cause of his symptom.

Only after several interviews with both the patient and his wife did I learn that just prior to the onset of the symptom, they had agreed to refrain from any form of sexual relations—and this was at the wife's insistence! She had previously indulged in sex only out of a sense of obligation and in order to have a family. Now that she felt she had fulfilled her part of the bargain, she wanted to call it quits. Being very naïve at the time, I could hardly believe my ears. Since then I have come to realize that many people do conclude their sexual activity long before nature intended. My patient said that he had made this bargain with his wife, not because he really wanted to, but simply in order to please her. Even the most radical proponents of women's liberation would recognize, I suspect, the utter absurdity of such an arrangement. My patient's condition began to improve as he was gradually able to assert his masculinity and face the real issues involved. However, it was no simple task to help him do so. Without psychiatric help to guide him, I doubt if he ever would have acknowledged the psychological basis of his symptom.

Another example of the way physical symptoms express and conceal serious emotional conflicts is that of a twenty-three-year-old girl who complained of weakness and occasional paralysis of her right arm. Medical and neurological evaluations were negative, and she was referred for psychiatric consulation. During the first interview, she was able to recall the circumstances under which her symptoms began. She had been looking at a picture of her mother, who had recently passed away. Just prior to the death, the patient had had a serious disagreement with her mother, in the course of which she had become so angry that for a very brief moment she considered picking up a knife and killing her mother. When her mother died shortly thereafter, the patient developed tremendous feelings of guilt because of her murderous rage, as if somehow she had been responsible for her mother's death.

This is a classic example of one form of pathological grief reaction where a part of the body, in this case, the arm, symbolically represents the murderous wish toward the lost loved one. Such problems are easily resolved psychiatrically by helping the person to remember the specific traumatic events associated with the death and to relive all of the emotions connected with it.

PREPSYCHOTIC STATE OF MIND

In addition to the kinds of symptoms previously described, there is another set of complaints that must be regarded even more seriously. I have chosen to call these symptoms "prepsychotic"; if not treated promptly and expertly, they are apt to progress to the point of actual psychosis. The trick is to recognize the prepsychotic state, for the symptoms are much more illusory and difficult to pin down. The patient feels that he is losing his mind, or the control of certain impulses. Specific bizarre feelings over-take him and threaten his whole concept of himself as a separate human being able to control his basic functions. His confidence is so shaken by the symptoms that he doesn't know from one minute to the next who he is or whether his behavior is suddenly going to change into something so radically different that he will lose his identity. Such a patient is never certain what is happening to him; he can't describe his feelings very clearly. He just had a constant foreboding, a constant uneasiness and premonition that his grip on things is slipping away.

Most patients who finally end up in mental hospitals, being labeled schizophrenic and other fancy terms, have probably been tormented by such feelings for a considerable time before finally acknowledging the need for treatment. Many of them still won't recognize the problem even after some interested friend or relative encourages them to get help. Unfortunately, by the time some people actually do become psychotic, they are no longer aware of being disturbed, because of illness itself becomes a solution to the intense discomfort that preceded it. It's not unusual for a patient in the throes of acute psychosis to tell you that he has finally figured it all out and that he knows all of the answers to life's problems. When someone tells you this, beware! He has probably organized a very unreal, if not delusional, system of beliefs as a substitute for the tremendous psychological pain he has been suffering. The prepsychotic state is a very unstable one. If treated adequately, it can be helped rather quickly. If ignored, however, it can rapidly deteriorate.

I detected that one young lady was in just such a fluid phase. She was a very attractive, intelligent, popular, recent college graduate from a stable family background. That, ironically, was her main trouble. Her life had always been so highly structured for her that when she was turned loose in the real world, without being adequately prepared to care for herself, she began to decompensate. She complained of feeling disconnected, of having a sense of "nobodyness." This feeling persisted for minutes or days at a time, always accompanied by a sense of emptiness and depression that caused her to become panicky. At these times, it seemed to her as though she was not actually participating in life but was merely a bystander who was observing her own behavior. On the other hand, these sensations did not significantly interfere with her normal functioning and she was able to hold down a job as well as attend to her housekeeping chores.

The prepsychotic states can all be grouped under the general heading of depersonalization, which means essentially that the sense of self is disconnected from the sense of functioning in the everyday world. A discontinuity appears between the two elements. More than any other state, perhaps, this condition requires immediate competent psychiatric attention and should never be taken lightly. It is no passing phase that will gradually disappear of its own accord. When a person begins feeling out of focus with himself or with reality in general, this is the very quintessence of needing a psychiatrist. A psychological life literally hangs in the balance. There has already been too much procrastination; to postpone things further would be equivalent to an act of psychological suicide. Interesting to note is the fact that this young lady, encouraged by her parents, had always been a model child. She had played the role of the perfect little girl, always doing the right thing and never betraying any genuine emotion—only a superficial kind of pleasure with anything and everything. On the surface, she had always been extremely popular, had shown above-average leadership, and had even been president of the student body. Through it all, however, she had never developed a true sense of her own identity except in relation to the structured environment of home and school. The result was an altered mental state that threatened to become psychotic.

A FULL-BLOWN PSYCHOSIS

People need a psychiatrist long before they become raving maniacs. By the time a patient becomes psychotic, the problems have mushroomed to the point where they are much more difficult to treat. This is one aspect of being a psychiatrist that is so very frustrating—over and over again, we see patients who have become horribly isolated from the real world and we know that treatment two or three years earlier could have prevented such a pathetic outcome. We probably could have saved them if only someone, anyone, had taken it upon himself to guide the patient into competent hands. So many families and friends compound the frustration when they tell me that Uncle Charlie had always been a little strange, so they figured he was just being himself and that there was no reason to be seriously concerned. They waited until he blew his mind completely, and then they couldn't get to a psychiatrist fast enough.

I met up with Uncle Charlie while I was still a resident in Boston. He was sixty-five years old and a bachelor, but still going strong—wine, women, and even a very important executive position. He had always had his little "eccentricities." He wore outlandish clothes, would never eat at another person's home, and never liked being far from a telephone. Shortly before his breakdown, he he began to drink more heavily and seem somewhat withdrawn. He complained about the fact that his latest girlfriend was uncooperative. No one paid much attention to him, however, until he walked into the local constabularly and told them he was turning himself in for stealing money from various collection boxes.

Strange as it may seem, he had reported such behavior, both to his boss and assorted friends. They had merely told him that he must be working too hard and to go home and take it easy for awhile. Charlie tried this, but he couldn't forget; he was too sick. He locked all the doors and windows and barricaded his apartment against the imagined onslaught of the FBI. When his brother arrived, Charlie slipped him, spy fashion, through the door and refused to speak English. Communicating only in his native German, on the assumption that the FBI would not understand him, he revealed a lengthy plot whereby government agents planned to persecute him for his misdeeds. The patient's brother was mystified by all of this, but it was only when it finally dawned on him that the poor guy was seriously ill that he finally convinced him to seek help.

Hollywood likes to depict psychotic patients frothing at the mouth and behaving wildly; but cases like that are virtually nonexistent. Psychotic patients can and frequently do exhibit bizarre behavior but frequently they go downhill so gradually, so insidiously that the people who know them most intimately are generally oblivious to the process that is unfolding before their eyes.

A thirty-two-year-old business executive came in to see me about his wife. She was suing him for divorce because she believed he was a homosexual. He admitted being somewhat passive in his sexual relationship with her, but vigorously denied ever indulging in any kind of gay activity. He further stated that the more he tried to prove to his wife that he wasn't a queer, the more she believed he was.

This woman managed to convince her attorney that her husband was a full-blown pervert; she also convinced the family physician. A minister was equally taken in by her superficially convincing account. What she succeeded in doing, finally, was to create a self-fulfilling prophecy: her husband eventually was rendered sexually impotent by her crass accusations. He was so bewildered by her that he felt castrated. Further, he could not turn to his lawyer, his doctor, or his minister. Like the majority of people today, he apparently did not realize that many psychotic patients can be perfectly sane and rational in all other respects and still be grossly out of touch in one specific area. The wife was able to discuss all aspects of her life with complete clarity and logic—until it came to the matter of her husband's suspected homosexuality. Her delusional thinking was limited to this one subject, and unless you pursued the question with her, you'd swear she was entirely rational.

In retrospect, two important things emerged from this case. First, the wife had begun being suspicious of her husband many years prior to the suit for divorce. Had he paid sufficient attention to her suspicion when it first began, psychotherapy would have been much more effective. Second, the woman had been seen by another shrink before she consulted me, and he had advised involuntary commitment. As it developed in my treatment of this case, such a move would have created a major focus for this woman to have become fixated on her delusional ideas and might possibly have led to the spread of her psychosis into other areas of her mental functioning such that she might never have been discharged. Doctors, lawyers, clergymen, and psychiatrists are all vulnerable. They certainly are not infallible. In complex cases like this one, it is frequently desirable to get more than one opinion before pushing the panic button and invoking commitment procedures.

Psychosis is not usually so difficult to recognize. Most psychotic patients become so overtly confused that even a child could spot it. They're unable to function in their primary roles as housekeeper, parent, breadwinner, soldier, or whatever the case may be. They lose the ability to concentrate and their relationships with other people break down. Their behavior becomes disorganized and reflects the inner turmoil from which they suffer. The loss of contact with reality that frequently accompanies this condition makes it necessary that a relative or friend assume the responsibility of seeing that the patient gets adequate help. Too often, however, other people are reluctant to assume this responsibility. They refuse to face facts and admit that the husband or wife or friend is mentally ill. Despite our so-called enlightenment, the phony assumption still persists in this country, much to the detriment of its victims, that mental illness is something to be ashamed of, as if mental illness were the same as being possessed by devils.

It was only by the grace of God that one woman didn't lose her husband in a traffic accident on the busy Capitol Beltway surrounding Washington, D.C. For twenty years, she had refused to admit that his increasing agitation and secretiveness were indicators of mental illness and not just a reluctance to confide in her. This man, for most of his adult life while pumping gas and fixing flats in a small-town service station, harbored the conviction that he had been chosen by his country to perform some special function. He did not know what mission he would be called upon to perform, but every time he saw certain newspaper articles or imagined that someone was following him, he was convinced that the Secret Service was trying to communicate with him in some unknown fashion. After twenty years of waiting, he finally decided to make the trip to the FBI headquarters in Washington, D.C. to find out the exact nature of his assignment. When officials at the FBI office told him to go home because his name did not appear on their list of special agents, he became acutely disturbed. He stopped several times to turn around in the busy Beltway traffic. Incredibly, he managed to find his way home, but he was in such a state when he arrived that even his wife was finally forced to acknowledge how very sick he was.

Relatives and friends play a very important role in the treatment of the psychotic patient. Even if the illness hasn't directly intruded upon all family members, the very presence of this type of illness in one member arouses reactions in those around him. Such reactions must be brought out into the open and resolved. The role that a patient's relatives must assume is that of supportive understanding of the problem, learning how to help him cope with it, avoiding emotional confrontations that might aggravate the problem, and helping to meet his responsibilities for him until he is in a position to assume them himself.

BEHAVIOR DISORDER

In no category of emotional disturbance is the role of the family more important than in that of patients with behavioral disturbances. These are the people, who through their disturbed behavior, are constantly causing grief for others and getting themselves into trouble. This category includes the addict, the sex pervert, and the antisocial character. They essentially set up their own rules for living—rules that are in sharp conflict with conventional standards. They don't care about the consequences of their actions.

There are many kinds and degrees of addiction. All addicts need psychiatric treatment, but most of them are unwilling or unable to follow through. Even when the patient himself is not well motivated for treatment the family invariably needs some counseling in order to effectively handle the addict. The family members must learn where to draw the line in their efforts to help the addict as well as how to draw the line.

If you know someone who is literally poisoning himself with cheap gin or heroin or LSD or some other toxic substance, go ahead and knock yourself out getting him help, but if he doesn't respond to your efforts—stop! Wait for him to make the next move. Don't foster a pathological dependency upon yourself that will only contribute further to his habit. Once you realize that the person in question is not going to listen to you, no matter what you say or do, unless he is committable on the basis of being an immediate danger to himself or others, get the hell out of the picture and let him fend for himself. Let him sink all the way to the bottom because, frequently, it's only when an addict hits rock bottom that he finally decides to get the help he needs. If you get to him before this—before he becomes properly motivated, you only set yourself up for being exploited, perhaps to the extent that your own mental health is jeopardized. Talk the situation over with a competent psychiatrist, and he will help you draw the line in the most constructive way. By avoiding a premature commitment to the patient, you avoid complicating your relationship with him to the point where you may well end up rejecting him completely. The strategy here is to keep the door open and yet not invite him in until he wants to come in.

"But he is going to kill himself," one distraught mother told me about her eighteen-year-old son who was a speed freak. No addict really wants to kill himself and, unless there is an accident, will stop short of that point. However, if he is completely rejected by his family or if his family does not set very definite limits on what they will tolerate, he is more apt to reach suicidal proportions. In the former case, it is because he feels completely rejected and in the latter, because he does not fully understand the limits—another psychological tightrope that the family has to walk with the psychiatrist.

The families of criminals and sex deviates likewise need psychiatric counseling. There are many techniques to help patients in situations like this; the friends and relatives need to be told what they are and how to apply them in the given case. The competent psychiatrist can help the relatives deal with any of their own problems that may have been stirred up by the deviant behavior. He can also advise them on how to relate to the patient without allowing their own hang-ups to complicate things. These behavioral disorders create many difficult problems, and the average family has no way of knowing what to do about them. Talking to a minister or family doctor does not usually do that much good. The people involved need to talk with someone with whom they can go all the way about their feelings, confusion and sense of inadequacy.

HOW TO KNOW WHEN A PSYCHIATRIST IS NEEDED

This question of who really needs a psychiatrist in some ways poses quite a dilemma. It's so easy these days to look around at some of the excuses for humanity springing up—bearded, barefooted wonders of the younger generation, sleek and perfumed money-mad symbols of the establishment, or the eccentric recluse down the street who throws stones at the kids when they come too close to his home—and decide that everyone around needs a psychiatrist. You have to be fairly cautious. Just because someone's life style isn't the same as your own, just because he disagrees with your convictions or prefers a different set of values does not mean that he is mentally deranged. Even when a person begins to behave abnormally, and theoretically might need a psychiatrist, it doesn't always imply that he will accept or benefit from treatment.

You don't just impose psychiatry on people because they are not everything you would like them to be. Sexual deviation is a case in point. If you approach a well-adjusted homosexual and say, "You've got a problem, baby, and you need help," he's going to laugh in your face. He might even tell you that you're the one who needs a headshrinker, and he might be right. Many people whose behavior reaches criminal proportions are satisfield with themselves as they are. Since they are not hurting psychologically, it's silly to pressure them into seeing a psychiatrist. They must be in serious conflict about their behavior, in terms of the effects it has on other people as well as on themselves, before they are motivated to seek help.

WHAT THE DIFFERENT PSYCHIATRISTS DO ABOUT RELATIVES

One of the traditions of psychoanalysis, which has outlived its usefulness, has been to exclude all of the patient's relatives from the treatment, as if the patient could be isolated from his family in any real sense. Unfortunately, psychiatrists have, in the main, continued this kind of isolationism, overstressing the privacy of individual treatment. They argue that what goes on between therapist and patient is strictly confidential, that the patient has to work out his problems on his own, and that the family would only contaminate the work that has to be done. Though there is some truth in this, it overlooks the fact that such isolationism frequently tends to complicate the patient's problems because it promotes resentment and confusion among the other family members, thus placing additional stress on the patient.

Today's competent psychiatrist not only recognizes the importance of responding properly to the questions of key relatives but also includes the latter when necessary in the treatment. This does not mean that he betrays anyone's confidence; he usually checks with the patient in advance so that he or she fully understands that nothing is going on between family and therapist behind his back. In selected cases, he will do family therapy, treating all members as a group simultaneously.

The Imitation Analyst would rather be caught dead than talking to any of his patient's relatives. The Doktor and Good Joe types might be willing to answer simple questions but usually don't do so in ways that facilitate the treatment. If a patient's husband calls the Doktor to ask how he can be helpful in his wife's treatment, he's apt to be put off with, "Don't worry about her; she's coming along fine. Just see that she takes her medication and keeps her appointments." He's really telling her husband to get lost and not take up his time with phone calls. Aside from the fact that his prediction might be all wet the Doktor has missed an invaluable opportunity to find out more about the patient and her problems.

Under similar circumstances, the Competent Psychiatrist would probably invite the husband to come in and discuss the whole situation. In this way he might learn the essential ingredients of the patient's behavior outside the office. He might also discover ways in which the husband is contributing to the patient's illness.

The Problem Psychiatrist regards the patient's relatives as enemies. In his tendency to overidentify with patients, he projects most of the blame for their troubles onto the relatives, thereby completely alienating them and cutting off what is frequently one of the most useful adjuncts of treatment. The Swinger is prone to do likewise. The Pigeon-Holer might not actually alienate the relatives but he is unable to make therapeutic connections between the categories in which he puts the relatives and those in which he has pigeonholed his patients.

The Organizer simply palms the relatives off on the nearest social worker. Social workers have a valuable place in psychotherapy, but when a competent psychiatrist calls one in to treat a relative, he maintains constant communications about the case and continues his own work with the patient on a regular basis. When the Organizer turns a case over to a social worker, that's it baby, the patient has probably seen the last of his psychiatrist.

Very few life problems requiring psychiatric intervention do not also require some attention to other family members, though maybe in a very peripheral way. I have interviewed boy friends, girl friends, husbands, wives, parents, even distant relatives at times. Frequently a patient's children have to be seen so that their role in relation to the problems can be fully understood. It is not unusual to discover that the children require as much individual help as the patient. Family therapy, in which one or more members of the immediate family are included in sessions with the patient, has become increasingly popular in recent years. Some misguided shrinks, however, have jumped on this bandwagon to the extent that they make family therapy a routine procedure in all cases without accurately identifying the specific needs of the patient and discriminating adequately between those who do and those who do not require this form of therapy. The Swinger type is apt to be seduced in this direction.

It becomes necessary to give attention to key family members when dealing with that patient group suffering the various symptoms of anxiety, depression, and psychosomatic reactions. After the patient's underlying conflicts have been exposed, the members of the family will frequently be required as part of the total treatment. For instance, if a woman's main hang-up is associated with her husband's recent tendency to be more critical of her, the competent psychiatrist will want to interview the husband as soon as possible in order to assess the total relationship. He will want to discern if the husband is projecting his own problems onto his wife. If it turns out to be one of those cases where hubby won't even come in to discuss the situation, then the psychiatrist has to treat the patient individually. He would prefer, however, to treat both members in accordance with the requirements of the situation. The treatment can frequently be expedited in this way.

In prepsychotic cases, it is frequently helpful to have other family members fill in background details that the patient himself might not recall. In the case of psychotic patients, it is not only helpful but frequently necessary that relatives provide a complete background history and be counseled themselves. (I have already mentioned the role of key relatives in the behavior disorders.) This becomes even more crucial when one realizes that patients with these afflictions frequently do not tell the whole truth and, in some cases, lie so compulsively that the psychiatrist may never be able to get a straight story without outside assistance. Drug addicts are particularly notorious in this respect and will conceal even from each other the latest bits of antisocial behavior. Junkies are so unreliable that the therapist needs as much leverage as he can get—through the family and other sources such as the probation department—in order to confront the patient adequately with the implications of his behavior. For it is only by doing so that the therapist can tap the patient's motivation and get him to acknowledge his need for change. These principles also apply in treating alcoholism, sexual deviation, and other forms of psycho-pathy.

Believe it or not, it's possible to have a relative attempt to sabotage the patient's treatment. One mother made repeated calls to tell me that her daughter, my patient, kept complaining that nothing was being accomplished in her treatment. At the same time, she threatened her daughter, telling her that the treatment would be discontinued if the daughter did not conform her behavior to the mother's own unrealistic expectations. I lucked out on that situation because shortly after the girl started in therapy, the parents were divorced and father assumed custody. Had this not happened, the therapy would have been doomed. No other relative in the picture was strong enough to control the mother's behavior. She was a real demon who had been in psychiatric treatment herself for years without significant improvement.

Another archenemy of the psychiatrist is the relative who, in order to feel superior, actually needs the patient sick. This type will try to involve the psychiatrist in heated discussions about the patient's behavior every time the patient begins to assert himself in a more healthy way. The wife of one of my patients once threatened to sue me because she felt I was encouraging him to be too independent of her. I wished her and her attorney luck, and from that point on, she never bugged me again.

Fortunately, most relatives do not have a vested interest in perpetuating the patient's illness. The situation, however, does occur with appalling frequency, and it contributes, perhaps more than any other factor, to the premature graying of the psychiatrist. If anything, though, too many friends and relatives are overly reluctant to call the psychiatrist, even when the patient's behavior is verging on the suicidal. To avoid meddling, they refrain from speaking with the therapist about very important matters. Some suicides could be prevented if people were not so fearful of being meddlesome. Are you your brother's keeper? In this very vital area, you are.

If you are a friend or relative who is vitally concerned about the patient's welfare, feel free to call the therapist to discuss either the background of the patient's illness or his current functioning. If the illness is a severe one, prepsychotic or psychotic, you should not hesitate to ask the psychiatrist about any problems affecting your relationship with the patient so that you will be better prepared to cope with the situation. Many problems come up in the course of any psychotherapy, and the patient usually benefits from the discussions.

In one case, the husband of a schizophrenic patient suddenly decided to withdraw her checking privileges because he felt she was spending too much money. He did this without consulting either me or his wife; this led to a significant deterioration in her condition. She felt that she was being treated less and less as a human being, and whenever she felt this way, her condition would get worse. Had the husband let me in on his decision, together we could have avoided this further trauma to his wife.

Another potential source of conflict between the patient and his spouse is whether he should drive while he is on medication. This needs to be discussed with the psychiatrist. Difficulties arise when a patient withdraws sexually from his spouse for varying periods. There are no hard and fast solutions for any of these problems; each case must be decided on its own merits. No decision of any magnitude should be reached without first consulting the patient's doctor. Many psychiatrists will shrink from the open invitation that I have extended to all concerned friends and relatives. The last thing they want is to be harassed by additional phone calls—even though their patient's life may depend on it. We don't need these sanctimonious bastards in the field—who tend to isolate themselves both from the families of their patients and the world of reality.

PSYCHOTHERAPY FROM OTHERS BESIDES PSYCHIATRISTS

The field of mental health has a broad spectrum of workers, many of whom are quite competent in psychotherapy. If you need psychiatric help and your problem is not too difficult, the competent psychiatrist may refer you to a psychiatric social worker, a clinical psychologist, or a psychiatric nurse, causing you less expense and sparing the doctor's limited time. As a matter of fact, most inpatient problems are diagnosed and treated through the team effort of a psychiatrist, a social worker, a psychologist, and one or more psychiatric nurses, thus permitting adequate coordination of the disciplines. Which member of the team actually carries the brunt of the treatment is not important as long as he is qualified, knows his limitations, and consults with the psychiatrist when the need arises.

Outpatients, except those in public clinics, are less apt to be treated by members of the ancillary professions. Very few psychiatrists in private practice have a working association with a social worker or psychologist; they prefer to handle their entire case loads by themselves. In the occasional clinic (like my own), which does make use of a team approach, the psychiatrist sees and evaluates each patient before deciding on the best therapist for that individual. If he assigns the case to someone else for therapy, he continues to supervise the treatment even though his personal contact with the patient may be limited to writing a prescription or evaluating physical symptoms. This, of course, is the obvious solution to the manpower shortage in psychiatry today; too few shrinks, however, know how to employ the method so that it is advantageous to all parties concerned.

If you, or anyone you know, is in need of psychiatric help, the sooner it is obtained, the better. Don't allow yourself to procrastinate for any reason. If you have a life problem, get help for it now before it becomes a full-blown neurotic illness. If you have psychosomatic symptoms find out why before they become chronic and you turn into a hypochondriac. If depersonalization is your problem, seek teatment before your condition mushrooms into a psychosis. There is no doubt about it—if everyone beginning to have difficulties received treatment within a few weeks of the onset of their symptoms, there would be no such thing as chronic schizophrenia in this country! (This assumes, of course, that they all received competent psychiatric help.) Think of all the hospital beds, currently tied up, that could be used for more constructive purposes. All the state hospitals devoted to the custodial care of the chronically ill could be shut down. Do you realize what I am saying? Early treatment or preventive treatment could virtually eliminate most of the mental illness plaguing America today. If you have a problem, it's your responsibility to seek and find competent professional treatment. If you are on drugs, wake up and get the help you need. If you are a friend or relative of someone with problems, then do your part to encourage him to seek the help he needs. The sanity you save will be your own—and your family's.

WHEN DOES A CHILD NEED HELP?

When a youngster needs a psychiatrist, and I refer now to children under the age of thirteen, there are some special factors that must be considered. First of all, children with emotional problems tend to react to them in a much simpler way. Although they can at times develop rather elaborate psychiatric symptoms, most of them react by not doing what is expected of them and rebelling in one form or another; they become "naughty." Some children will develop psychotic symptoms. The vast majority, however, will merely act out their conflicts with behavior that is more infantile than one would expect of a child that age. It may be bed wetting, hair pulling, setting fires, or disruptive classroom behavior.

When a child becomes frustrated, he usually does something to someone in order to seek relief from his underlying feelings. Parents are, therefore, apt to react to his behavior by disciplining him rather than by seeking competent psychiatric help. So, if your child or any other child close to you, begins acting "badly," despite the fact that his behavior up to that time has generally been quite acceptable, ask yourself if, perhaps, he isn't reacting to a build-up of internal tensions before you resort to strictly punitive measures. Since children are not as psychologically sophisticated as adults, they express their conflicts in more primitive ways. Furthermore, it is when the child does not respond to the usual punitive techniques that psychiatric evaluation may be necessary.

Being a parent is probably the most difficult job in the world. Dealing with children takes native ability, good training in one's own childhood, and a lot of experience; it doesn't just come naturally. (If it did, we psychiatrists would have a hell of a lighter case load.) Parents also have to be in tune with the times, more so today, perhaps, than ever before since values and traditions are changing so rapidly. Even the experts are writing books on child rearing that conflict sharply from one year to the next—Doctors Spock and Ginott notwithstanding. Nothing in our educational system prepares people for the role of parent. They have to pick up little bits and pieces along the way and pray to God they will work. Usually they don't discover until it's too late, that they didn't make it with their kids after all, that something is wrong in their relationship with them and that the children may seriously need outside help.

When seeking help for their disturbed children, parents encounter a unique phenomenon—the child psychiatrist. For some reason, which I have not yet been able to determine, it was decided many years ago to set up a separate specialty of child psychiatry. The child psychiatrists are required to take four years of psychiatric residency training instead of the usual three, and two of those four years are devoted to work with children. This was an unfortunate development, because it tends to make something special of the fact that children may need psychiatric help as well as adults. It leads to parents being able to scapegoat their children as being the sick ones who need help. Such parents will try to absolve themselves of all responsibility in the matter since it is the child who is showing the disturbed behavior and not them. This tends to promote the false assumption that the child is the patient and that the parents are really well. Nothing could be further from the truth.

When we deal with disturbed children, we are dealing with a disturbed family unit. To regard the matter in any other way simply does not do justice to the realities involved. The child is very dependent upon his parents and is an integral part of the total family scene far beyond puberty. Those two residency years devoted exclusively to working with children are intended to help the psychiatrist learn to work intensively in psychotherapy with the kids—no matter what the family problem or how incidental it may be that the child is the one showing symptoms. The whole family is usually the real patient.

How can the real patient stand up when the child psychiatrist is focusing primarily upon the disturbed behavior of the child himself?

I do not recommend, therefore, that you look for a child psychiatrist when the need arises. Rather, I would suggest you seek out a competent general psychiatrist with whom to discuss the problem. If he then feels that consulation with a child psychiatrist is necessary, let him make the referral. Do not assume, when Johnnie begins shoplifting and defying parental authority, that you automatically need the services of a child psychiatrist. It may be some adult problem at home to which he is reacting.

Many parents, however, are so loaded with guilt feelings about their child's behavior that they will do almost anything to avoid seeking competent psychiatric advice and treatment. Should they feel guilty? All parents of children under thirteen should feel at least partly responsible for their child's behavior. The amount of actual responsibility or guilt in the production of the child's symptoms, however, will vary considerably from one case to another. At one extreme, you have the whole range of disturbances caused by child beating, neglect, and abuse all the way to the more subtle forms of psychological torture inflicted so proficiently by some emotionally ill-equipped parents. In such cases, it is certainly the parents who need treatment more than the children. If they receive the necessary help, the children will fall into line.

At the opposite extreme, where parental responsibility may be minimal, are the children who have certain unique inborn characteristics that tend to make them stand out from their peers. Children can be different in many ways; they can be intelligent, retarded, short, tall, sensitive, creative, hyperkinetic, physically handicapped, brain damaged, etc. It is extremely important in such cases to correct any physical deformities that may be leading to psychological problems. When they can't be corrected and when the child as well as the parents are unduly distressed by them, they have become psychiatric problems, and consultation should be obtained as soon as possible. The longer one delays, the greater the chance the child will develop a psychiatric complex about the way in which he is different from other kids his age. To be sure, some children can be very cruel toward anyone who stands out from the group. The parents may simply not know how to handle the situation.

Precocious or delayed sexual development is always a potential source of psychological problems, and when parents cannot deal with these matters as they arise, they need psychiatric help. In such cases, the parent of the same sex as the child needs to be involved in the treatment since a child identifies sexually with that parent. Mother may be more aware of the problem, but father must become involved with his son's hang-ups. When a disturbed boy is brought to me, I will insist on seeing his father as well as his mother. If he is frequently out of town on business, I will wait until he is in town to see him. Too many fathers are allowed to get away with this kind of nonsense.

In between the two extremes previously mentioned are the children who get hung up on some specific childhood fear or tension. Growing up is never an easy process, and, along the way, children experience just about every fear known to man. What happens is that the child experiences a specific fear, let's say the fear of death, for example, and it will correlate in turn with a specific fear that one of the parents may have. Neurotic reverberations are set up between the parent and child so that what was initially a simple aspect of psychological development mushrooms into a psychological complex. The parent is not really to blame for the way he or she has intensified the problem; but, if the parent receives the help needed and can then apply this to the child under expert psychiatric guidance, the child himself never really has to be a patient. As a matter of fact, with every adult patient I see who is married and has children, I am indirectly treating the children as well. You can see why I am not a fervent believer in the specialty of child psychiatry.

Children have an innate tendency to grow up normally if given sufficient psychological room and guidance by their parents. So many parents, despite everything that has been written on the subject, continue to cause problems by focusing excessive attention on one aspect of their child's physiology—giving enemas, making the child eat, fussing about masturbation, making a boy into the little girl they want or vice versa—in other words, imposing their own frustrations onto the child.

Whenever a parent has particular difficulty relating to a specific child, that parent needs a psychiatrist. It is not unusual to have a child that you just don't respond to in the same way that you respond to your other children. This does not mean that you are a bad parent who should feel guilty because you don't always love this child. It may mean only that you cannot be all things to all people and do need some psychiatric guidance so that you can learn how to tune in to this specific child's basic psychologic needs in a way that you were unable to do previously. Some children simply have temperaments that are so much the opposite of their parents that the latter actually feel helpless in their relationship with the child.

Adolescence, or the early puberty years through the late teens, has always been a period of intense emotional arousal. The child's instinctual demands are being felt very strongly. His thought processes are leaping beyond the limits of family tradition. He is desperately trying to find a meaningful role for himself in his society. The residual conflicts that the parents may have in relation to themselves or the world in general are always enhanced by the aroused state of the average teen-ager. Because of the radical transformation our society is undergoing at the present time and the early exposure our teen-age children are getting to excesses of sexual promiscuity, drugs, riot mongers, and violence, many parents of teen-agers can benefit from psychiatric consulation. The parents who have a definite feeling of being unable to keep up with their children in today's changing world stand to benefit from consultation with a competent psychiatrist.

It is the rare parent today who feels he is completely in control where his teen-age children are concerned, or who can bridge the generation gap successfully enough to maintain an open system of communication with them. However, most parents are not fully awake to the existing crises and, therefore, don't recognize their need for help. Hence they do not readily seek competent professional guidance before the situation explodes. By the time most parents come to me, the child has already run away from home or has become addicted or has attempted suicide or is about to become a parent prematurely. When things have been allowed to go this far, the kids themselves have frequently gone beyond the point of wanting help. They have built up a resentment toward people in positions of authority and regard psychiatrists merely as spokesmen for the establishment and, therefore, inherently evil.

Many psychiatrists have unwittingly fallen into the trap of siding with the establishment and making conformity their basic principle for guiding human behavior.

Or they have gone to the opposite extreme and sided with the rebellion of the younger generation against the establishment. Thus, they are unable to define their role clearly or appropriately enough to be able to meet the needs of either the parents or the children. The competent psychiatrist does not choose sides in these matters. On the one hand, he recognizes that many of our society's traditions are outmoded. He realizes that much of what parades under the guise of relevance is mere hocus-pocus. He senses in today's politicians a Machiavellian pragmatism that is bound to demoralize the aspirations of youth. He sees in the structure and functioning of most school systems a kind of rote classroom procedure and dehumanization that turn the students off rather than awaken their intellectual and involved curiosity. He sees further the ways in which parental frustrations and conflicts in so many families also turn children off and stir up their dissatisfactions with the establishment.

On the other hand, the competent psychiatrist is aware that many adolescents today are so hung up on their rebellion that they shut off all positive, constructive channels of communication. Through meaningful identification, he sympathizes with parents who have struggled for years to provide reasonable limits and controls for their floundering children, only to have them broken down by social indifference and the permissive trend of the times. He realizes also that the "do your own thing" fad has been terribly exploited by some members of the younger generation, much to their own detriment. In other words, by pursuing a pain-free and pleasure-seeking existence, they betray some of the higher achievement goals, passed down through the centuries, that could contribute to the betterment of man, if more young people would pursue them.

Parents of adolescents need to get in touch with a psychiatrist at the very first sign of trouble. Don't wait until your son impregnates a young girl, despite the fact that the abortion laws have been liberalized. Don't wait until your kid takes an overdose of drugs or has a bad trip on LSD. Don't wait until he leaves home in an impulsive rage. Alert parents can detect signs of difficulty long before these things come to pass. As soon as you realize that your teen-ager's behavior is threatening to get out of control, seek competent psychiatric counseling; it is not too late to salvage your child. It will be too late if you hesitate because of false pride or because you think it is too expensive or because you simply feel that things like that are not supposed to happen in your family.

Teen-agers on drugs need a psychiatrist as much as anyone does. I have never interviewed a junkie kid who did not have multiple family problems as well as an underlying core of depression. Since drugs are primarily an escape mechanism for today's rebellious youth, all parents must be aware of the possibilities involved since drugs are so readily available. Kids who are fairly healthy don't need to escape as desperately and, as a rule, don't really get hooked, though they may experiment temporarily. It is when the adolescent has significant problems to start with that drugs are apt to become a way of life for him. Like a gal told me in the office the other day, "That's all I look forward to, using drugs, and you want to take that away from me."

Of course, there is a lot of experimentation with drugs going on, trying the forbidden just because it is forbidden. You and I did it when we secretly smoked a few cigarettes, and when we drank a few beers before our parents really approved. Yes, it is true that the pushers are taking advantage of this. However, the kids who get hooked, the kids who become so addicted there is no way to approach them without professional help, are the ones who had adjustment and emotional problems in the first place.

The answer to the problem, once an addiction has been established, lies in a combined psychiatric and correctional approach. A psychiatrist alone usually cannot control a junkie kid. When he reaches that point, he simply will not listen to anyone else unless he has to. No matter how well meaning friends, relatives, or parents may be, they just aren't going to get to first base with the kid. As a matter of fact, trying to communicate with such sons or daughters, after they have already turned you off and tuned you out, is like pouring salt on the wounds. It only alienates them further and hardens their resistance. If parents have been too rigid, have not set adequate limits, or have been inconsistent in the raising of their children, when the children reach adolescence, all hell will break loose. The parents need professional help long before things reach this point.

Getting hooked on drugs is the final stage in a long history of emotional struggle. The law may well impose penalties that are too severe for possession of marijuana, but only the law, in many cases, can stop a kid from going all the way. Mental health professionals and people in the department of corrections, particularly the probation officers, are simply going to have to work together more effectively than they ever have before. The lawyers who defend these kids are also going to have to do more than just try to cop a plea on the basis of having referred their clients for psychiatric treatment. They also will have to assume greater responsiblity in the actual rehabilitation process. Merely preventing a kid from going to jail does him no good at all if he is back on the streets within twenty-four hours looking for his next fix.

For parents to get their money's worth out of psychiatry, they have to recognize both how they have been successful and how they have failed with their children. They have to be able to admit to themselves what their own strengths and weaknesses really are. They must be willing to learn how to improve their relationships with their kids. Many parents of disturbed children don't have the foggiest notion of what a healthy parent-child relationship is all about. Or, if they do, they are frequently compensating for an unhealthy marriage through their relationship with their kids. Though this is a less direct form of psychological exploitation, it is just as destructive to the child's growth and maturity. A competent psychiatrist can help any parent with problem children to become less of a problem himself. In the process, the child's problem will eventually be resolved.

WHY PEOPLE RESIST SEEING A PSYCHIATRIST

Estimates vary considerably, but I would guess that one out of every five people needs a psychiatrist. We know that all people who need psychotherapy aren't going to get it. They will refuse to accept the need for it in spite of all the obvious indications. Even some of those who recognize the need will be unable to go through with it due to various fears and misconceptions. Sometimes it's the family of the patient that expresses the heavy resistance.

The primary reason for this reluctance is still the stigma associated with psychiatry. Although in certain parts of the country seeing an analyst has become a status symbol, most of the nation still suffers from the fear of what other people might think. "Aunt Matilda would think this was the end of the world if she knew I was seeing you," remains a common refrain. Well, all I can say is,

"To hell with Aunt Matilda!" If she has such a hang-up, she may well need psychiatric treatment herself. If people were not so concerned about what other people think, twice as many people would probably get the help they need; and the Aunt Matildas of the world would become historical relics, pitied more than respected for their archaic views. To a certain extent, of course, when someone tells me how concerned he is about what other people might think, he is also talking about himself.

Everyone has the fantasy that he is in complete control of his own behavior. This is a fiction of the mind, a necessary working assumption for a person to maintain his sense of responsibility. Those patients who equate psychotherapy with losing control of their own behavior feel very threatened by it and have a stronger tendency to resist it. They feel that going to a shrink means that they are no longer in control. They seem unable to realize that the conscious decision to seek help when it is really indicated is a sign of much greater control than they generally exercise.

Similar are the patients who are fearful of becoming dependent upon anyone else. They are usually people who had to become overly independent at a very early age, and anything that threatens their continued state of pseudo-independence is quickly negated. They will go to excessive lengths to preserve their false feeling of independence; they rarely, if ever, ask for help. It's amazing how many doctors and nurses fall into this trap. They have grown so accustomed to feeling in complete control at all times that it is extremely difficult for them to assume the role of a patient. This is a corollary of what I said earlier about doctors going into medicine because of their fear of loss of control over life and death itself and psychiatrists choosing their specialty because of their fear of losing control of their own emotions.

Next, some people really feel that having to express any kind of emotion is the same as expressing weakness. More common in males, it reflects their desire to rise above all expression of human feeling. In our society, it is much easier for a woman to come in and talk about her feelings. Men, on the other hand, have been taught from early childhood to bury their feelings, to grit their teeth and bear the pain, that you're chicken if you cry or even express the frustrations that may have been gnawing at your guts for many years. From the psychosomatic point of view, the capacity to cry is probably the single most important and direct form of expression that we human beings have. It is so important that I find myself asking patients almost routinely, "When was the last time you remember crying?" The answers I get are almost routine, too. "Cry? Me? I never cry." Suddenly we are a nation of Indians. Expressing basic feelings for these people, seems to be some kind of a sin. Yet, it is very therapeutic.

The next resistance is money. People ask themselves what right headshrinkers have to make "so much money." These same people spend hundreds of dollars for simple surgical procedures, such as appendectomies or hernia repairs, without any qualms whatsoever. Emotional illness, which affects the very quality of the lives they lead, is in its own way, just as debilitating as physical illness— maybe more so. It certainly causes as much torment as does organic disease. If surgeons can make a couple of hundred dollars in half an hour removing an inflamed appendix, then good psychotherapy must be worth thousands of dollars an hour in terms of the skills, training, and results involved. I know of no other service in our community that is worth any more money, assuming it is competently performed. Nor do I know of any qualified man in the profession who won't cooperate in making individual financial arrangements when the patient requests it.

Then there are the people who resist psychiatry because, for one reason or another, they have had to keep their emotions bottled up all of their lives, and they are afraid of what might come out once they uncork them. They are little Pandoras who don't want to lift the lids of their psychological boxes for fear that terrible things will come pouring out and drive them crazy. Many people panic at the very idea of opening up to another human being; a few of them have some basis for their fear—especially if they place themselves in the hands of an incompetent psychiatrist. A psychiatrist must be able to pace his patients within their limits of safety. If patients, who have a huge reservoir of untapped emotions, are encouraged to open the flood gates too rapidly, they may not be able to cope with the overwhelming feelings involved. Like water suddenly breaking through a dam, their emotions may rupture the very tenuous hold on reality that they have maintained for many years. The competent psychiatrist, however, can spot a potential flood immediately. He doesn't rush the therapy but lets this type of patient go at his own pace. He doesn't probe deeply but chooses areas for discussion that can be comfortably handled. Many more people fear such an overwhelming emotional tide than actually are susceptible to it, but, nevertheless, this is one of the common resistances to psychotherapy.

Another common fear is that the psychiatrist can somehow read the patient's mind. Patients think that because he is known as a headshrinker, he knows what they're thinking before they know themselves—and they think there might be some things they would not want to reveal. Psychiatrists cannot read minds; they have no clear idea of what patients are thinking until they are actually told. They sometimes anticipate their patients and in doing so, get the implied meaning of the words before the patients themselves do. But that is the very reason you go to a psychiatrist: to have him listen closely to what you are saying, more closely than you are able to listen yourself, and tell you what he is hearing. If he seems at times to anticipate you, it's not because he is reading your mind but because he is getting the straight scoop from listening to you—he really hears you and must, if he is to provide you with the feedback necessary for you to understand yourself in a way that will promote constructive change on your part.

Another group of patients are like J.B., who had been turned off by psychiatrists themselves. Competent psychiatrists frequently have to contend with and undo the mistakes of their colleagues. They know all of the complaints by heart—and, hopefully, so do you by now. Psychiatrists are too medical; they're too cold, they're too personal; they're too eager to turn patients over to someone else. They either don't respond at all or they are overbearing; they keep patients coming back indefinitely without really helping them. I hear the same gripes repeatedly. It is unfortunate that psychiatrists themselves cause patients to resist psychiatry, but that's what happens when you get tangled up with the wrong guy.

Psychiatry is a branch of medicine, and it's helpful for potential patients to recognize that it is just as dangerous to treat emotional problems themselves as it is to treat physical ailments. Just as they would seek help for a broken leg or a bout of pneumonia, so should they for a bad case of nerves or an emotional hang-up. They need to realize that they cannot resolve their conflicts themselves and that only with the help of a skilled psychiatrist can they get better. Persons fearful of losing control, becoming dependent on the therapist, or exhibiting a show of weakness need to work through these anxieties with a competent therapist. They need to realize that, despite what some psychiatrists think of themselves, no headshrinker has supernatural powers. No psychiatrist is able to influence his patients in any way that is repulsive to them. As far as the social stigma is concerned, patients must recognize that their mental health is far more important than anyone else's opinion. If there are specific people about whom the patient is concerned, these feelings should be worked through thoroughly in the treatment.

In the face of extreme resistance to therapy, patients should be encouraged to see the psychiatrist once before finally making up their minds. It seems less threatening, somehow, for a person merely to meet a psychiatrist and talk things over than it does to anticipate weekly sessions over a long period of time. In many cases, a competent psychiatrist can resolve the resistance once the family gets the patient through the door. But not always! I remember one father practically twisting his schizophrenic daughter's arm to get her into my office, only to have her tear back out into the car within five minutes. There was nothing I could do to get the girl into treatment at that time. Nonetheless, I spent an hour with her father discussing ways in which he could gradually overcome her resistance.

One of the problems in this case was the father's overtolerance of her psychotic behavior. He was compensating for his own guilt feelings since he felt that his own marital problems and eventual divorce were largely responsible for his daughter's illness. He had assumed custody of the girl and, for a number of years, had tried to treat her himself rather than seek the kind of psychiatric treatment she really needed. Like so many parents of retarded children, he tried to alleviate his sense of guilt about the child by attempting to cure her himself rather than by doing what should have been done.

If the patient refuses to see a psychiatrist under any circumstances, then a member of the family should seek a consultation. The psychiatrist may suggest to him ways of handling the situation. I'm not saying that this will always solve the problem, but in many cases, the psychiatrist can recommend techniques that might work. Do not assume the situation is hopeless until you have really explored all the possibilities.

PSYCHIATRY IS NOT ALWAYS THE ANSWER

Psychiatry is not the answer to every problem. Although there are unquestionably psychological connotations attached to most problems—legal, financial, family, what have you—the need for assistance is indicated only when the psychological factors become dominant or pathological. Nevertheless, there are always instances of people misusing psychiatry—either for their own vested interests or because they don't really understand what a psychiatric problem is. We're back to the original question, "Do I have a problem or don't I?" In some cases they don't! At least not a psychiatric problem.

One of the best examples of this was a woman who complained of an obsessional fear that her husband was having an affair with their teen-age foster child. I examined the woman and didn't find much wrong with her. So I asked, "What makes you think your husband is *not* having an affair with this girl?" When I went into detail with her, some rather indirect evidence turned up indicating that he really was playing around with the girl. In fact, the evidence was more than suggestive, but the wife didn't want to believe it. I told her that before we went ahead and assumed she was delusional, she had better have a little talk with hubby and find out just what was going on. A few days later she called to tell me that it was true, that her husband had confessed to a sexual relationship with the girl, and that she was going to arrange for the child to live elsewhere.

The woman had a problem certainly, but it was a problem easily solved by getting the facts in the situation. As it stood at that point, the only psychiatric problem she had was her tendency to avoid asking the obvious question. If the woman's fears had been delusional then, yes, she would definitely have had a psychiatric problem. If in the future she should have problems reconciling with her husband or if the husband had been sexually frustrated because his wife was frigid, the couple would have required treatment. Had the foster child developed any conflicts over the affair, then she might have required treatment. As it turned out, however, all of the participants in this little drama were relatively healthy; they were able to handle the conflicts aroused without psychiatric intervention.

Another case I had was a hypnotist, an entertainer who wanted to take his wife to the annual hypnotists' convention on the west coast but was stymied because she wouldn't leave their three children with her mother. He called me late one night, saying, "Dr. Lazarus, I'll pay you any amount of money you ask, fifty dollars, a hundred dollars, anything, if you'll just answer one question for me." I knew there was something wrong right away because there aren't too many people willing to fork over a hundred bucks for a quick yes or no answer. I asked him what the problem was. He said his wife was afraid her mother wouldn't take as good care of the children as she did, and she was afraid something might happen to them. His question finally was, "Is it all right for my wife to go with me to the convention and leave the kids with her mother?" I needed some extra money at the time, but I couldn't prostitute myself that much. I said, "Look, this is a problem between you and your wife. Maybe she's being overprotective of the children and maybe she isn't. Since she feels so strongly about it, it would be silly for me to give you a yes or no answer."

Well, that's one instance when there was no need to call a psychiatrist, especially at his home late at night. You don't ever call a shrink and try to bribe him into siding with you against another member of your family. If you want your wife to go on a second honeymoon with you and she refuses, you've got to resolve that problem yourself. If you think that your wife's reasons are unsound and she needs psychiatric help, then go ahead and make an appointment for both you and your wife, but don't expect a simple yes or no answer to a loaded question. Even an incompetent shrink will spot this kind of manipulation and refuse to be sucked in.

The staff of a nursing home was also guilty of a similar abuse. I was asked to consult on an eighty-year-old man who was making passes at the attendants during his bath. There were no male attendants in the place, just female, and the guy would get so sexually stimulated while being scrubbed, he'd expose himself and try to seduce the gal bathing him. This stirred the hell out of the whole staff, so I agreed to see the old guy. He turned out to be pretty normal for a man his age; he had found a way to get an erection, and he thought that was the greatest. I felt he was only doing what came naturally and that the nursing home administrator needed help more than he did—since hiring a male attendant would have solved the problem immediately. Actually, I felt that the sexual stimulation was probably good for him, though I refrained from pointing this out. As it was, their inhibitions were being strained beyond comfortable limits. I limited my consultation to a few pointed remarks about the sexual attitudes of nursing home attendants and let it go at that. I heard nothing further about the case.

I could write a book on just the humorous cases I've seen. People sometimes get hung up on the damnedest things. Like the people who come in because their bridge partners are undergoing treatment, and they don't want to feel excluded. Or the women who come in because they've gained ten pounds and have heard that anyone who is overweight needs psychotherapy. True, some fat people have emotional problems that cause them to overeat, and they're not going to be able to hold their weight in check until they get them resolved. No psychiatrist, however, can cure the average case of middle-age spread. No psychiatrist can tell an old man that his days of wine and women are over when, obviously, they're not! No competent shrink is ever going to tell a guy how to handle his wife, unless they are both interviewed and the real problems are brought to the surface.

THE PREVENTIVE FUNCTION OF PSYCHIATRY

In addition to the segment of the population that really needs psychiatric help right now, there's another large group who would also benefit from such help. Despite there being no single, all-inclusive explanation of human behavior, despite the lack of good research and all the guesswork going on, we still know enough about human behavior to do a hell of a lot more than we're doing on the level of prevention. Anyone in a crisis situation can benefit from psychiatry. There are certain developmental phases in everyone's life that are definitely critical.

We have already noted that the way problems are handled in childhood can make or break the future adult.

Adolescence is an equally critical period. Most adolescents experience some turmoil; a kid at this stage in his life needs all the help he can get. Young adulthood suggests marriage and parenthood. There are very few people who decide to get married for logical reasons as well as the usual emotional ones. The skyrocketing divorce rate indicates just how many mistakes are being made—each divorce represents two people who have made bad decisions. Selecting a husband or wife is one of the most critical decisions a person has to make, and most would benefit from prior psychiatric consultation. Also, the kind of adjustment problems arising early in marriage can be dealt with quite readily if both parties are willing to try.

Becoming a parent is another crucial phase in the life cycle. Many young people do not have a healthy precedent on the basis of which to model their own behavior. They have only a little intuition and Doctor Spock to guide them, neither of which is very reliable. As children are going through their various developmental crises, the baffled parents would benefit greatly from talking with someone more familiar with child development. Some pediatricians are quite proficient at handling the routine kinds of problems, but the more serious ones, certainly, should be brought to the attention of a competent psychiatrist. One case in point is that of a mother who was terribly concerned about her daughter's masturbation. The pediatrician had told her merely to ignore it; the child would outgrow it. Mother, however, was unable to ignore it; she dwelled on it to the point where no amount of simple reassurance calmed her. Fortunately, she had the good sense to come in and discuss the whole situation openly. As it turned out, the masturbation problem was only one in a series of problems in the mother-daughter relationship. Pediatricians are a bit too fond of telling harassed parents that the child is going through just another phase, just as many internists are apt to tell a psychosomatic patient that it's all in his head and to go home and forget about it. Many people cannot and should not accept this superficial advice. They have feelings and conflicts about the problem that have to be resolved, and the psychiatrist is the man for the job.

A couple who realize that their marriage is in trouble should always discuss this with a competent psychiatrist. Divorce counseling, by the way, is just as important as marital counseling. From the point of view of the future mental health of the two parties involved, whether the marriage stays intact or terminates is a separate question. Prolonged legal battles for the custody of the children must be avoided at all cost. Though more wives today seem to be granting custody of the children to their ex-husbands, this should be accomplished without dragging the children through an extended court battle. Having seen many psychiatric casualties among the the children of such disasters, I can only say that parents who allow this to happen thereby prove their unfitness as parents.

The middle years are loaded with potentially depressive conflicts. Your life is half over and you begin to realize that you are running out of time. You wonder where the hell you've been all your life, where you're going and why. All the plans you make for retirement seem meaningless and empty. You are prone to dwell on the idea that life is just a farce, and you lose interest in things generally. Get thee to a competent shrink without further ado.

Elderly people, knowing that the end is approaching, are also susceptible to bouts of serious depression, particularly if they have not already put their psychological houses in order. When a person has not done so, the

minor organic changes associated with senile and arterio-
sclerotic brain disease can develop into pretty explosive
personality changes that require psychiatric treatment.
Just about anyone who is headed down the last lap would
benefit from talking out his worries, fears, and feelings
with a competent psychiatrist. The latter can offer elderly
patients ways to reconcile the past, enjoy the present, and
minimize the fear of the future.

A competent psychiatrist can also deal effectively
with the dying patient, which is an important and challenging task. Meeting death is more difficult than most
people care to realize. Death anxiety permeates all
psychiatric illness and, to a certain extent, all human
beings have to reconcile themselves to the inevitable.
The capacity to confront death in a rational and mature
fashion is probably the toughest thing any human being
is ever expected to do. Despite all of the emphasis lately
on sex education in the schools, I strongly believe that
it is even more important for death education to become
part of the regular curriculum. This whole area is so very
important that almost any family group who has lost a
member would profit from talking about the loss with a
psychiatrist. When the deceased is a wife or a husband,
the surviving spouse would benefit from such help, no
matter what state of emotional health existed before the
loss occurred.

Most people about to undergo major surgery would
benefit from talking with a competent psychiatrist. This
is particularly true for anyone undergoing an organ
transplant. Many of today's surgeons are well aware that
when the patient is particularly fearful about the proposed surgery, he often has an unfavorable postoperative
course. When open-heart surgery first became practical, it was noted that approximately one-third of all
patients undergoing this procedure developed a transient

postoperative delirium or psychosis. I conducted a study to find out if psychiatric consultation before surgery would reduce the incidence of these reactions and discovered that patients who were up tight or depressed about the surgery could be helped, psychologically, to deal with the situation. By instructing recovery room nurses to pay as much attention to personal factors as physical factors, the incidence of psychotic reactions following open-heart surgery was significantly reduced.

The same holds true for any type of surgical procedure. A patient's fear of death and anxieties about life always increase when he faces the prospect of a potentially fatal procedure. Although surgical fatalities have been dramatically reduced in recent years, the possibility is still there. The fear of being anesthetized, and thereby losing control temporarily, is also a relevant human consideration. Some patients equate this forced loss of consciousness with their fear of dying. Such patients would benefit from a brief period of psychotherapy prior to the actual procedure, in elective cases. In some cases, where psychiatry and surgery can cooperate fully with one another, the psychiatrist might even suggest that the surgery be postponed until the patient is better prepared psychologically to tolerate it. I have done this several times and feel strongly that the postoperative course was considerably improved by it. One prospective open-heart case was in therapy a full year before I was satisfied that he was psychologically ready to withstand the trauma of the operation. As a result, he recovered rapidly and without complications. This kind of teamwork between the two fields is rare, however. Surgeons generally don't like admitting other specialists into their private domain, least of all psychiatrists. Times are changing and if a patient is facing a simple hernia repair, hysterectomy, gall bladder removal, kidney transplant, or heart surgery, and is seriously frightened by the prospect, he or she would benefit from one or more sessions with a competent psychiatrist.

It isn't hard to realize that any chronic illness is going to have psychological effects on the patient. No matter what the illness—arthritis, emphysema, colitis, or paralysis secondary to a stroke—it is going to create certain obstacles in the former life style of the patient. In some ways, he might still be the same person, but, physically, he's no longer able to keep up. A good headshrinker can assist him through his ensuing depression and help him find a reasonable middle ground between his former capacities and his current limitations. Without sound counseling at the time of the illness or injury, patients are apt to add an emotional handicap to the physical one.

A fifty-year-old male patient I am currently treating is a perfect example. He fell from a scaffold, sustaining a moderate degree of brain injury that resulted in generalized weakness, some paralysis of his left side, and occasional epileptic seizures. He was unable to continue his lifelong work as a bricklayer. In fact, he was no longer permitted to drive a car. He had always had anxieties about being a good provider for his family, as well as some doubts about his masculinity. In addition, he harbored guilt feelings about certain traumatic events that had occurred much earlier in his life. These various emotional conflicts might never have come to a head if the accident had not occurred. As a result of his handicap, however, the conflicts became severely aggravated, and he developed a suicidal depression in the months following the accident. Had he received psychotherapy immediately after his injury, there probably would have been no need to hospitalize him two years later.

There are innumerable emotionally charged events that could be smoothed over with psychiatric assistance.

Pregnancy is one. It used to be thought that a pregnant woman shouldn't be treated psychiatrically because therapy might stir up too much anxiety and only complicate things. Now we know that nothing could be further from the truth. It's during pregnancy and childbirth that all of a woman's conflicts are stirred up. More than ever she can benefit from talking with a competent psychiatrist—one who knows enough about pregnant women to assess what's normal and what's not, what needs work and what doesn't. Such consultations would not only reduce the pregnant woman's fear of delivery and pain, but would reduce incidence and severity of postpartum depression as well.

Relocating is another crisis for many people, especially teen-agers. Our society has become so mobile that it is commonplace for families to be shifted around from one place to another. Though some people thrive on this transient kind of existence, others resent having to tear up their roots and say goodbye to old friends and familiar places. Kids who are juniors or seniors in high school have an especially hard time of it. They frequently have difficulty making new friends and become bitter about the transplant. In many instances, they don't understand the reasons for the move and blame their parents for their dissatisfaction.

When we talk about who needs a psychiatrist, the question really is, who doesn't need one at some time or other in his life. More people need psychiatric help today than ever before. There is more questioning of traditional values. Our society is so mobile there are few stable communities left. People expect more satisfaction today in terms of their own needs; women especially are on the move—no longer content merely to be maids to their husbands and children, reaching out for greater purpose and commitment. The actual violence in our society is a constant reminder of the potential violence within each of us. The various wars, declared and undeclared, that we have experienced have contributed to the increased restlessness of younger generations. The sexual revolution has created as many problems as it has solved. People don't have to work nearly as hard as they did fifty years ago; their lives aren't nearly as structured, and there's a lot more room for individual freedom and choice, creating more conflict in predisposed individuals. We are building increased amounts of dehumanization into our society—overcrowded classrooms, overcrowded ghettos, mass production, phony advertising, and emphasis on materialistic goals as measures of achievement. Individuality and self-esteem are being swallowed up by the demands for increased production and greater earnings. Creativity and pride of craftmanship have become lost arts. Where is the dividing line between dehumanization on a social level and depersonalization on an individual level?

Unfortunately, more people need help today than there are facilities available. Less than half of the people who need and want help will actually get it because of the relative scarcity of good psychiatric facilities. At this writing, there just aren't enough competent psychiatrists to go around. As I see it, the only answer is to practice preventive psychiatry: see more patients earlier in their illnesses before their problems become massive. Treat patients for shorter periods of time but give them better therapy during that time. Encourage people to consult a psychiatrist before they really need one!

CHAPTER **4**

Seek And Ye Shall Find

YOU HAVE NOW decided that you or some member of your family needs to see a psychiatrist. You are also now aware that all practitioners of psychotherapy are not equally competent, that many are not even capable of practicing minimal therapy, and that few will actually be able to meet your psychological needs. The imitation-analyst type will be inclined to extract from you certain preconceived notions that may make you worse than when you started. The medically oriented type will pin a label on you and tend to overdose you with pills and advice. The swinger type is going to try out his latest fad on you. If you are unfortunate enough to get a problem psychiatrist, then you're in real trouble; and the good Joe psychiatrist will love you until death do you part.

The selection of your psychiatrist is, therefore, one of the most important decisions you will make in your life. This is the guy you are going to bare your soul to right down to the very bone. This is the guy in whom you are going to place your confidence, your trust, the future state of your mental and emotional well being. This is the guy with whom you are going to struggle emotionally, harder than you've ever struggled in your life. What decision is more important? Making a business investment? Buying a home? Having another child? Simple decisions compared to this. How about choosing a mate? That's a tough one all right. I would equate the problem of selecting a psychiatrist with that of choosing a marriage partner. I cannot emphasize strongly enough the importance of selecting a competent psychiatrist—and the right psychiatrist for you.

How, then, do you go about locating a psychiatrist in your community, one who can relate well to you and your life situation and understand your particular hang-ups? Do you go to your priest or rabbi? Do you consult your family doctor or the local medical society or perhaps talk to a friend who is currently undergoing therapy and accept a layman's view of the whole profession?

DO NOTS

First of all, do not go to the first psychiatrist that your friend, neighbor, or even close relative recommends. People have a tendency to seek out a shrink who is a member of their local church or country club. Their ignorance about the profession and their insecurity, resulting from their anxiety or depression, leads them to seek some phony kinship with the therapist. But, face facts! A psychiatrist's ability to treat you, or anyone else for that matter, depends on how talented he is at his job, not on his religious affiliation, his social standing in the community, his prowess on the golf course, what model sports car he drives, or what style shirts he wears.

Neither should you go to your clergyman for advice. Many clergymen are convinced that psychiatry is great, psychology is great, the various ancillary professions are great; they even practice a little amateur stuff themselves. But they still don't know who to refer you to because there just isn't that much interaction between the church and psychiatry—the two go their own ways. That isn't the way it should be, but unfortunately that's the way it is; so it is best not to mix religion and psychiatry in terms of selecting a therapist.

Do not consult the local county medical society. The best they will do is give you the names of three psychiatrists in your area, at least two of whom are not very busy and can thus take on new patients, and the third, probably a name the receptionist happens to remember for no good reason at all. County medical societies make no effort to discriminate between doctors and, of course, it would be inappropriate for them to do so professionally; neither do they offer you anything but statistical and educational information about the names they give you. They even asked me, in my early years, if I wanted referrals despite the fact that they knew very little about me or the kind of psychiatry I practiced or whether I was able to help my patients. A medical school diploma and psychiatric residency training are all that matters to them.

Do not contact a private or public mental hospital or the psychiatric department of a medical school for help. If you call a private hospital, you will have to request a specific person, and who are you going to ask for? The secretary or the medical director? A psychologist or the chief social worker? The medical director, himself, is a psychiatrist but not necessarily a competent one; therefore, if you put yourself in his hands, you may be licked before you start. The psychologists and social workers at a private hospital have certain commitments to the psychiatrists on the staff and are involved in their own petty politics, so they cannot be completely objective with you. State mental hospitals are not much better; they are little worlds unto themselves, isolated from the community at large. Personnel at these institutions are apt to turn you off with, "We don't make such recommendations. We're too busy with our own patients.

I ruled out medical schools because they have a very strong bias in favor of the teaching psychiatrists. I was heavily committed to teaching for seven years and have no objection to teaching, but there's no reason to believe that teaching makes a guy a better practitioner or even a good judge of those who excel among his colleagues. There are politics involved here, too. Many medical school psychiatry departments are partly financed through the private practices of their teaching doctors. So, naturally the chairman of any of these departments will refer you to one of his boys to keep the funds coming in. If you know of a medical school so well funded that it is in no way dependent of revenues from private practice, you might get some knowledgeable answers to your questions there. Few schools today are in that enviable position and, in fact, chairmanships of psychiatry are currently going begging because of the financial situation.

As a matter of fact, do not seek advice about the selection of a psychiatrist from anyone who happens to be a shrink himself. Even if you know him personally, and you think he might level with you, your best information will come from a different source. Don't bother to contact your local branch of the National Mental Health Association. Primarily a fund raising organization, the Mental Health Association is more or less under the thumb of the county medical society and will simply refer you back there for another random three names.

If you think I'm being too hard on the establishment, let me tell you what happened when I made some anonymous calls to these agencies in my own community. The

County Medical Society gave me three names. (I wasn't surprised!) One was a Good Joe Psychiatrist, one was a Problem Psychiatrist, and the third had been in town less than five months, so no one really knew anything about him. I didn't bother with the hospitals because I'm entrenched enough there to know that route by heart. The secretary in the psychiatry department of the medical school—I never did get through to the head of the department—gave me another three names. You guessed it—all teaching shrinks in the medical school. And the gal at the Mental Health Association, in purring voice, referred me to the county medical society—would I like the number? In other words, every one of these organizations did exactly what I had predicted they would do.

Do not select a psychiatrist on the basis of how famous he is, how much publicity he receives, how many best-selling books or technical articles he has published, how prosperous his waiting room looks, or how many times he has appeared on television. These factors are no more relevant to you and your problem than his religion, his political preferences, how handsome he is, or how sexually potent he may be. Finally, do not give up in desperation. In spite of any impression I have given you to the contrary, psychiatry does, in fact, remain a viable field of medicine and you, or anyone who cares to, can seek and find a competent psychiatrist.

THE DO'S

Basically, there are two valid approaches to seeking and finding a good headshrinker.

The first one is to consult your family doctor—if you are lucky enough to have one and have confidence in him. Unfortunately, the general practitioner, or family doctor, is a vanishing breed, as is the warm, personal knowledgeable, doctor-patient relationship that went along with him. However, it still exists in some areas, usually among older generation physicians. Where it does exist, patients have the advantage of really knowing their doctor, his strengths as well as his weaknesses; and they can truly evaluate and rely on his opinion. After all, this is the guy who pulls them through their worst illnesses, sits up nights with them, and works hard to keep them well.

Assuming, then, that you have a family doctor, by all means ask him to refer you to a competent psychiatrist. If he gives you an answer such as, "Well, my experience has been that most shrinks need a psychiatrist themselves" or "Don't waste your time and money going that route—they won't do you any good," you will have to discount his advice as unreliable because he is strongly biased against psychiatry. He may have good reasons for his prejudice.

After all, what I'm telling you is that many shrinks aren't worth going to; they will only take your time and money and give you nothing in return. I'm also saying that there are some good psychiatrists, too, and if you need one, it is your responsibility to find a competent one. Don't create hard feelings with your family doctor, but don't let him deter you from getting the help you need. Ask him if he would have any objections to your proceeding anyway. Usually he will tell you to go ahead if you want to. It may well turn out that the relationship you develop with your psychiatrist will become just as important to you as the one you have with your family doctor.

Many general practitioners, however, respect the field of psychiatry and have had some experience with specific psychiatrists. If your doctor counters with the fact that he really does not know much about the local psychiatrists though he has referred a few patients to

Dr. X, then you should immediately ask, "What was the outcome of those patients?" Don't be reluctant or embarrassed to ask this question. It is entirely relevant, and from his response you can assess the amount of confidence he has in that particular person. He may say, "Well, one of them got better, but another didn't," which means he's not too enthusiastic about this guy. He might tell you, "The majority of patients I have referred to him have improved," which shows he has a good bit of confidence in the man. He may suggest that he has been very good with certain kinds of problems but hasn't gotten to first base with others, indicating that he has fairly good insight into the psychiatrist's overall capabilities. In this case you will, of course, ask him if your problem is one that this specific psychiatrist is capable of dealing with and, if not, if he knows of another who would be better able to handle it.

You might really luck out and get an answer such as, "Well, there's Dr. Y. I've referred a number of patients to him, and most of them have gotten better." If you get a straight and unequivocal answer like that from your family doctor, then you have it made. You are now on the royal road to a good psychiatrist. This man has met the needs of your personal physician who has referred cases to him and gotten good results. The mark of the competent psychiatrist is consistent, favorable results. Unfortunately, there aren't that many competent psychiatrists, nor, as a matter of fact is there sufficient communication between psychiatrists and other doctors. If there were, competent psychiatrists would be more fully used and the incompetents would fall by the wayside.

In the event that you don't have a family doctor or that your physician is antipsychiatry, you will have to use a second approach for finding your psychiatrist. In this approach, you contact your local public mental health center and ask to talk with a psychiatric social worker who can advise you. Although you will eventually become a private patient, it is more feasible for you to contact a public clinic for information because there are fewer politics involved here. The personnel are usually familiar with local psychiatric treatment, and the administrator himself is frequently a social worker or psychologist rather than a psychiatrist. Thus he has more freedom to express his opinion about the psychiatric community. If the administrator is himself a psychiatrist, don't talk to him about the problem! He may be moonlighting and suggest you see him personally. Don't fall for that crap. Talk to someone else and avoid a hassle. It is too probable that he is an organization-type shrink, and as such, should be avoided.

It would be better to talk with the administrator in person, but if he insists on limiting you to a telephone conversation, then accept this as better than nothing. If possible, make an appointment to see him, saying that you want to talk about a psychiatric referral, that you don't want to entrust yourself or some member of your family to just any headshrinker who happens to be around, that you want some one capable of dealing with your particular problem, and that you would appreciate his taking the time to discuss the matter with you. His response may range all the way from, "No, I don't have the time" to "I'd be glad to;" he may simply offer you another three names. I don't know what the hell good three names are as opposed to ten names as opposed to one name but, unfair as it is to a patient, that's the standard procedure and may be the best that's available to you.

Most people connected with public clinics try to be accommodating, and you will probably get an affirmative answer such as, "I'll be happy to discuss it with you." The administrator may actually be surprised at your request, recognizing the intelligence of your decision to discuss the matter with someone who is familiar with the psychiatric community and the kinds of therapy being practiced. Most public clinic people are well aware that good therapy is scarce and will admit privately that there are only a few good psychiatrists in the average community. They won't admit it to you—a layman coming in asking for help—but as a visiting member of the profession, I can sometimes elicit their candid opinions. I'll ask them, "Are there any decent shrinks in this town?" And they'll look at me as if to ask, "How did you know that most of them are no good?" Of course, I know because I have practiced in a number of communities and visited in a good many more—and the situation is the same all over. Nevertheless, administrators look at me as if I were a spy from somewhere, checking up on them for the psychiatric society. They become slightly paranoid when someone talks that straight to them. Therefore, when you approach your administrator or social work supervisor, you must do it diplomatically.

Don't expect to get an immediate answer because he has to be very cautious about what he tells you; he has to protect his position in the community. The director of a public health clinic doesn't want you to go out and tell other people that he said Dr. Z was the only good head-shrinker around. This will reflect on him and his whole clinic operation. In no time he'll have every psychiatrist in town on his neck. You want to be careful, therefore, not to put this guy on the spot, yet still get the information you need from him.

When you arrive for your appointment, you might begin by saying, "I don't want you to give me any names yet. I want to tell you a little about the problem first; then you can tell me which of the many qualified psychiatrists in this town will best be able to handle it." In this way you are giving him lots of leeway but also plenty of reason to give you a specific name. If you want to pursue it even further you might ask one or more of

the following questions: Is he, the administrator, cogni-
zant of the general psychiatric community, especially
the psychiatrists who have private offices, and the kinds
of practices they have—psychoanalytic versus supportive
therapy versus whatever brand of psychiatry they practice?
Does the guy he recommends emphasize group therapy,
or is he more individually oriented? Is he able to wrestle
through the problems of his individual patients as well
as deal with any family pathology involved? Did this
doctor go into psychiatry directly after his internship
or did he drift into it later? Guys who end up in psychiatry at a later date, for one reason or another, never seem
to make the grade. They tend to become the medically
oriented type and have great difficulty readjusting to the
more flexible approach of the competent psychiatrist.
They probably went into psychiatry in order to cut down
on the long hours they had been working as G.P.'s but
still maintain their standard of living.

I also contacted my local, state-supported, public
mental health center while I was making calls. The first
time around, I was turned over to a psychiatric social
worker in the screening and evaluation clinic. This gal
was less structured in her answers and more sympathetic
than any of the other agency people. She gave me five
names—the five shrinks associated in some way with the
mental health center. I forgave her that one. After all,
those were the doctors with whose work she was most
familiar.

Most good psychiatrists will connect themselves in
a teaching or supervisory capacity to a public health facility. This is an indication, in itself, that these men feel
comfortable with all classes of people and are capable
of handling a wide range of problems—though some may
be no damn good with your particular hang-up. I then
gave this gal a specific problem and asked which of the

five could best handle it, but she would not commit herself beyond the five names, assuring me that each was
equally competent to handle any problem. Since I knew
all five shrinks (one was myself!), I knew that this was not
true, although I had to agree that collectively, they were
above the average in our locale.

The second time around, I held out for the administrator in charge of psychiatric services and ended up with
the medical director. This particular clinic was undergoing some changes in organization and, at the time I
called, the medical director was also acting as the administrator. My conversation with him was not satisfactory
because he, a psychiatrist, had offered to treat me in his
private practice. If you should run into a similar situation,
don't waste his time and yours. Instead, insist on speaking
to one of the nonpsychiatrists—a psychologist or social
worker—in a supervisory position.

If for some reason, neither of these approaches works
for you, there is one other alternative. Though I advised
you earlier not to go to just any psychiatrist recommended
by a friend or relative, if someone you know and respect
has personally consulted a psychiatrist and has gotten
good results, then certainly you should explore this possibility. If it doesn't seem as if your friend has benefited
from the therapy as much as he claims, don't be entirely
discouraged because, as an outsider, you may not know
the whole story of his initial problems. Your friend may
have made tremendous strides in an area you know nothing about. So go ahead and ask him about his therapist.
Ask him if the guy really helped him. Ask him if he would
recommend him to other people. If he answers "yes"
to both questions, then zero in on why he thinks the guy
is such a good psychiatrist. If the friend answers something like, "Well, he was really marvy," or "He seemed
like a real friendly person," then forget it. But if he gives

you some salient reasons, if he says, "Well, the guy really helped me when I was hurting, you know? He didn't only get me over my symptoms, but he helped me to achieve a greater self-understanding," then you'd better sit up and take notice. If you're still not absolutely positive, dig a little deeper. Put the same questions to your friend that you put to your family doctor or the mental health administrator.

Friends are always willing to pass around free advice; they can steer you wrong a lot of times. When they've had the benefit of experience, however, and know what they're talking about, the probability is greater that they are giving you a push in the right direction. If by chance your friend refers you to the same guy the doctor and the administrator recommended, then grab a telephone and make an appointment fast. Obviously this shrink is the popular choice, so popular he may be booked up for months, and you'll be lucky to squeeze your problems through his door within the next six weeks.

MATCHING PATIENT WITH PSYCHIATRIST

By now you have done the most important thing. You have accepted the fact that a wide spectrum of competency exists among practicing psychiatrists, and you have learned how you, a layman, can differentiate between the good and bad shrinks practicing in your area. As a result of your efforts, you have acquired the name of at least one competent psychiatrist and you are ready to place yourself in his care. There is still one more factor to be considered—especially if you are one of those fortunate ones who has acquired several names and now must choose among them. How do you go about making the best selection among competent psychiatrists?

Some time ago Harry Stack Sullivan pointed out how important it is to get the right mesh between patient and psychiatrist. Many factors can influence the compatibility that develops in the doctor-patient relationship, such as a common cultural framework, the doctor's expertise in certain areas, religion, sex, age, money—the list is endless. Let's take the socioeconomic factor. Most psychiatrists come from middle- or upper-class backgrounds. Others, like myself, come from the wrong side of the tracks. Patients, of course, represent all backgrounds, and the competent psychiatrist must learn to relate to these backgrounds, no matter how foreign or unlike his own.

Initially I had some difficulty relating to very wealthy patients. I remember one nineteen-year-old boy who stunned me when he told me of his wealth. He was a millionaire from a multimillionaire family, and most of his problems stemmed from money. One of his hang-ups was believing that people cared for him only because of his money. Another was fear of the degeneracy that so much wealth had caused in other members of his family. He was determined that it wouldn't happen to him, but in the back of his mind was the fear that it just might. I had never realized just how difficult the situation can become when you can spend only a small fraction of the annual interest on your capital and still live like a king.

When he first came in, I had a great deal of trouble relating to him. I grew up in a ghetto area of Boston where money was scarce and luxuries nonexistent. I couldn't imagine what it was like to have enough money, much less more than enough. I encouraged this boy to go to school and he tried—first art and then psychology, but both courses proved too dull for him. Finally, in order to learn the construction industry, he took a job as a laborer. He would stop by my office on the way home from work, covered with dust and dirt and looking like a peasant. Well, since I'm a peasant at heart, I found it easy to relate to this laborer, money or no money, and we resolved his problems in short order.

I have other wealthy patients who are more difficult for me. They are spoiled rotten, have maids and chauffeurs, and live the kind of life that I basically do not respect. In spite of that (or maybe because of it), I am able to help them. They begin to realize what phony lives they are leading, lives that are only perpetuating their problems, and are able to discuss their entire situations with me after a while.

Cases at the other extreme can be just as tough. One couple came in initially because of difficulties they were having over finances. They were in a financial bind all right, but that was the least of their problems. She was a beautiful, intelligent, shapely, twenty-six-year-old white woman who had been a call girl, very much in demand before her marriage. He was a tall, handsome, rugged, Negro chap, light-skinned and reminiscent of Harry Belafonte in appearance, but with not too much on the ball upstairs.

When I first saw the couple, the husband was holding down a menial job in the postal service and was on the lowest pay scale for civil servants. As if that weren't bad enough, he threw most of it away every payday shooting craps or laying it on the dogs. To make ends meet, his wife had begun entertaining some of her former clients who were delighted to have her back in business again. This infuriated the husband, who was basically a pretty straight guy despite the gambling. The situation had resulted in some violent emotional eruptions, which hadn't been helped any be neighbors and in-laws who rejected the couple rather forcefully, either on the basis of their mixed marriage or her former occupation.

Actually the two of them probably would have split up without ever seeking psychiatric help had she not suddenly become pregnant. But instead of smoothing things over the way they had hoped, the baby only added to their problems. Because he was jet black with kinky hair and flat features, the wife was having a hell of a time accepting her child. On top of it all were her guilt feelings for marrying him, his guilt feelings for marrying her, her near nymphomanic sex drive and dissatisfaction with the straight life, and his overbearing possessiveness and compulsive gambling instincts. It made for quite a case. The wife will require long-term therapy, and since he's not motivated for treatment, I'm not sure we'll ever get the husband straightened out. There probably aren't very many psychiatrists around who would even try to solve this kind of tangle. The majority of shrinks in this country wouldn't even know what to do if they wanted to be helpful.

A competent psychiatrist can relate to anybody from any socioeconomic group, from any cultural background, from any religious background—and separate the wheat from the chaff. But, damn, it's a hard thing to do, and most psychiatrists can't do it. So, if there is a unique social or ethnic problem of this sort in the patient, then it is even more important to be selective in choosing a psychiatrist. If one out of five shrinks is really good, it's probably only one out of ten who could adequately handle all the circumstances involved in the unusual case.

Another factor is expertise. There are not only levels of competence in psychiatry, there are also different kinds of competence. Some shrinks are better with problems than others. Some are very good at handling hysterical women with certain sexual hang-ups but when confronted with an aggressive male, who can only express his hostility and anxiety in occasional fits of temper, they run for cover.

Over the years I have acquired a certain expertise with psychosomatic problems. Another guy might work well with homosexuals. I am very critical of this tendency to subspecialize within the field of psychiatry. Any competent psychiatrist can cope with a drug addict; any competent psychiatrist can handle the psychotic patient. Nevertheless, if your problem is not of a conventional type—neurosis, anxiety, phobia, depression, psychosis—but involves one of the character deviations, then it is doubly important to check out the ability of your psychiatrist in that particular area. Ask your family doctor or public mental health center administrator if the shrink he is recommending is equipped to deal specifically with your kind of problem. Don't ask another psychiatrist. Most of them won't even admit that they do better with one kind of patient than another. It's that old conspiracy of silence among physicians, more so among psychiatrists than among other specialists.

The religious affiliation of either patient or psychiatrist should not be a significant factor, but there are always exceptions. The first question some patients ask are "Are you Catholic?" "Are you Jewish?" Are you Protestant?" At the time, it's very important to them. In a sound relationship between patient and psychiatrist, these silly hang-ups melt away as the patient begins to appreciate his own humanity, to recognize both his shortcomings and his strengths, and to evaluate the human struggle for what it really is. Once a patient has experienced this degree of insight, it's psychologically impossible for him to be prejudiced against anyone—and in good psychotherapy such insight is experienced more intensely than ever before.

Unfortunately, in much of what's called psychotherapy today, it doesn't happen. Therefore, to avoid additional problems, if a patient is extremely orthodox, is so hung up on religion, and leads such a narrow life that he feels uncomfortable with people of other faiths, then he should be treated by a therapist of his own faith. In direct opposition, if a person from a rigid religious background is rebelling against the religion, and this is contributing to his conflicts, then he should not see a therapist of that particular faith.

The religious hang-up can crop up in patients of all faiths. There are Jewish patients who can't possibly relate to a non-Jewish psychiatrist, and there are Jewish patients who should not be seen by a Jewish shrink. Very strict Catholics sometimes have trouble relating to a non-Catholic. Others treat the shrink as a priest, occasionally even calling him "Father." It's helpful when this happens because it gives the psychiatrist an opportunity to point out the differences between the two—and there are more differences than similarities. The whole concept of Catholicism raises a certain ambiguity, in view of the position the Church has taken in the past toward psychiatry. Psychiatry was considered a direct threat to the idea of the confessional: no secular agent of any sort had a right to so much information about a person's inner feelings; highly personal subjects, such as human conflicts and disturbances, should only be discussed with the priest in the confessional box. These matters were strictly between a person and his God; and the priest, as mediator, was the only one who had a right to this sort of knowledge. Younger generation priests tend to be more psychiatrically oriented than their older colleagues.

It is also the case that some psychiatrists harbor certain unconscious religious hang-ups—in spite of their residency training. I have heard Gentile psychiatrists discussing Jewish patients in a way that clearly indicated not only their biased attitude but, even worse, that they were unaware of it. I also know shrinks from narrow

Protestant backgrounds, who are so rigid that they can't handle certain clinical issues. The doctrine of original sin carries over into their thinking to the extent that they regard any expression of hostility as neurotic. What they really mean is that anger is evil and sinful; rather than tolerate anger from their patients and deal with the real conflicts involved, they gloss it all over with so much love and tenderness that the patients repress the source of anger even further. How can you tell one of these jokers, no matter how nice he is, that sometimes you feel like killing your boss or raping your secretary. That's evil; it's taboo! Patients soon learn what they can and can't talk about; of course, they shouldn't be talking to these psychiatrists at all. The Good Joe means well, but he allows the wounds to fester beneath the surface. The poison may then spread rapidly, and the patient suicides before Joe even knows what has happened.

Fundamentally, human problems are the same regardless of race, creed, or what have you. The competent psychiatrist can relate adequately to any religion, because his job is not to impose a code of behavior on patients, but to help them work out their own moral frameworks and develop their own sets of values in order to resolve their individual conflicts. Values, per se, are changing rapidly in our society, and headshrinkers are often identified with the more permissive attitudes and the looser moral climate—a layman's assumption that is not necessarily true. In any event, a shrink's personal values, other than his own humanity, should not enter into his work at all. The primary purpose of the psychiatric residency is to get rid of this tendency towards moral judgment. If a patient feels that his psychiatrist is judging him, then he had better look elsewhere.

Still another factor is the age of the psychiatrist. I'm not suggesting that there is any ideal age, but it is obvious in some cases, that a very young or very old psychiatrist is not appropriate. In most cases, the age range of thirty-five to fifty-five is satisfactory. If the shrink is much older or much younger than that, you'd better wonder, if perhaps, age is a crucial factor.

I remember one patient calling the clinic and asking for a "young, modern-thinking-type psychiatrist." As it turned out, she was wise in her request, because she was doing all kinds of things that many older-generation shrinks would have been unable to tolerate. They would have disapproved of her behavior, to the extent of losing their objectivity. A psychiatrist's disapproval can be an important factor with patients who are rebelling against parents and authority, experimenting with drugs, and questioning the values of our society. Older-generation psychiatrists frequently can't handle these problems. Many younger shrinks can't treat them either because they're too hung up themselves with the very same problems and can't remain neutral, which brings us back to the idea of competency again. I would not go so far as to suggest that only older psychiatrists treat older patients and younger psychiatrists treat younger patients. To the contrary, my experience indicates that older patients often prefer younger doctors, finding them more refreshing; and some younger patients find more security in older men. Anyway, those are some of the considerations concerning age.

Sex is another factor. There is a general tendency for men to have better results with women and women with men. I do have more difficulty treating males than females, the opposite of which is true for female psychiatrists. Freud was right about some things! Unfortunately, we don't have enough female shrinks. While I was teaching, I developed a special program to enable married female doctors to participate in psychiatric residency training by arranging schedules so that they could raise their families and still serve in the program on a half-time basis. This isn't done frequently enough, and we're not getting a sufficient number of women into the field.

The idea of opposite sexes being easier to treat works for homosexuals as well as heterosexuals. There is more natural rivalry between male and male than there is between male and female, although it can get pretty sticky between male and female too. It is especially appropriate, theoretically, for a patient in an acute homosexual panic (panic based on the fear of losing control of homosexual impulses) to be treated by a member of the opposite sex. If a young male is brought into the clinic in a homosexual panic of psychotic proportions, a female psychiatrist is far less threatening to him at that point than a male psychiatrist would be—unless he is a competent psychiatrist. I have dealt with many homosexual panics and they have gone fairly well, but I immediately structure the situation so that the patient recognizes quite clearly that there is no sexual threat involved—no chance, no possibility. I make this understood nonverbally more than verbally.

I do the same thing with females. I frequently have to point out to the female patient who is hung up on the big shot psychiatrist with seemingly all the answers, that there is no question here of any sexual relationship. Patients find this quite reassuring if the statement is timed properly. If, on the other hand, the shrink makes such a statement before a patient is ready for it, he deserves to lose the patient—and usually does. I can recall only one patient I lost under these circumstances, a nymphomaniac who was apparently determined to seduce me, just as she had compulsively seduced every man she had ever known. The psychiatrist must be warm and responsive to his patients' needs, it's true; but there are limits, and it's up to the psychiatrist to define them.

Every time a shrink becomes sexually involved with one of his patients, the whole profession suffers because of it.

Fees are something else to consider. You should find out about the charge in advance. Fees vary from one community to another, but you should find out what the going rate is in your area; then be sure the guy you've selected is in line with it. Be suspicious if his fees are either too high or too low. One is as bad as the other. If he charges less than the average, the obvious question is whether he tends to be self-depreciatory. You want a man who knows his own worth. Also, you should learn whether he schedules half-hour as well as full hour appointments and if he would be willing to make a financial arrangement with you in the event that you cannot pay his entire fee at one time.

Does he have any obvious hang-ups? Certainly shrinks have their problems. They can be just as neurotic as some of their patients. But if the hang-up is obvious, then stay away. In the course of your therapy, it's bound to become a complication factor. Does he hide behind an authoritarian front, medically speaking? Or, in other words, is he the Doktor type mentioned in Chapter 2, or any of the types other than the Competent Psychiatrist? If he is, by all means discard him—unless, for some unique reason, you would prefer your therapy to be skewed in a particular direction.

I have presented some of the more important factors that can influence the relationship you will form with your psychiatrist. If, in view of your problems, you consider the factors that seem important, and come up with one psychiatrist who seems to fill all the qualifications, then you're finally ready to consult the man of your choice. Don't rule out the possible need to switch later on. In spite of all your research, the competent psychiatrist you have selected may not turn out to be the one for you after all.

IN AN EMERGENCY

If Aunt Minnie, who has been noticeably depressed in recent months, becomes inconsolable and threatens to blow her brains out, do you panic and throw the gun away? If Johnny, whom you didn't know was on drugs, suddenly develops his own imaginary devils during a bad acid trip, do you call the police and report him for the illegal use of drugs? If you discover Uncle Filbert terrified and hiding in his room because the FBI is out to get him, do you tell him that the government is not that interested in his case?

The answer to these questions is obviously, no.

In an emergency, you must get the disturbed person to a psychiatric hospital as quickly as possible. Most people caught in an emergency situation know absolutely nothing about the psychiatric hospitals in their community. Our mobile society—the fact that people just don't stay very long in one place—probably contributes to this, but the real offender is more likely the stigma attached to mental illness. People just don't want to believe that psychiatric emergencies can strike them or their families. Consequently, when they do strike, people don't know where to turn, and they tend to panic. In an emergency situation, choosing the right psychiatrist is more difficult because there isn't as much time to consider all of the factors involved.

As in any other field, private treatment is preferable to public. Public hospitals, with their chronic problems of too many patients and too few staff members, are primarily custodial or holding operations. Public patients are medicated and occasionally, in the better institutions, given some group therapy. For the most part, however, they are herded around like a bunch of sheep. In private hospitals, patients are treated more as individuals; their therapy is frequently on a one-to-one basis and every effort is made to help them get well as soon as possible. It is true that some private hospitals give patients too much attention, but this is decidedly preferable to too little or no attention at all.

The question, then, of public or private facilities is one of finance. Does the patient have adequate insurance or sufficient personal funds to pay the bill at a private facility? Surprisingly few people seem to know whether their hospital insurance covers psychiatric confinement and to what extent. They go to great extremes to protect themselves against medical emergencies, but here again, they just don't want to think about mental illness. Mental illness won't ever happen to them. It only happens to the other guy—that oddball down the street. It not only can but does happen, and when it does, they are never prepared for it. It is not unusual for a patient to be admitted to a private hospital only to find out later that his insurance doesn't provide adequate coverage. In such cases the patient then has to be transferred to a public facility; this change can be detrimental to the treatment process.

If you are really concerned about Aunt Minnie or Johnny or Uncle Filbert, you should use any techniques at your disposal to get them into a hospital immediately. In emergency situations, you have the right to prompt and efficient professional service. You're the one who's paying for it, either in direct fees or, in the case of the public facility, indirectly through taxes. You should feel free to exercise whatever pressures that can be brought to bear on the situation. The only tenable obstacle you may encounter is the unavailability of a bed. There is still a gross shortage of psychiatric beds in many communities and, although steps are being taken to remedy this situation, you may be forced to accept some kind of temporary help until a bed does become available in the hospital of your choice.

Let's say it is 1:00 A.M. when all hell breaks loose. The patient may be playing with a loaded revolver or returning from a midnight stroll brought on by the need to track down his pursuers. Go through the very same process that I have outlined above in the nonemergency situation. This time, however, abbreviate your inquiry. Don't keep the family doctor on the phone for more than ten or fifteen minutes at such an ungodly hour. Ask him whom he recommends, whether that man conducts a hospital practice, and why he selects him rather than anyone else. If his answers make sense, don't prolong matters. If they don't, call the emergency service of your local mental health center, assuming they have someone on call at night. He may not relish having his sleep interrupted but when his head clears, ask him the same three questions.

If neither approach works, call the emergency room of your general hospital, inquire about the local mental hospitals, and then call the hospital directly. If you have not been able to establish contact with a specific psychiatrist by this time, the doctor on call that night will handle your case. In the event that he gives you a lot of static, as does happen frequently at that hour, or he tells you to wait until 9:00 A.M. when the admissions office opens, tell him exactly what you think of him. If he does not relent, call another hospital and repeat the process. Hopefully your patient will sign in voluntarily. If not, after discussion with the psychiatrist, decide whether you or some member of the family should sign an order for emergency detention that very night.

Above all, don't let the hospital's red tape get you down. Keep your cool, no matter what—the situation is already explosive, and your getting up tight will only complicate matters. Do what you have to do at the time the emergency arises. The next day is soon enough to investigate the situation in more depth. If you find later on that you would prefer a different psychiatrist, you have every right to switch doctors. Unless you request a change, however, the psychiatrist on call will probably assume full responsibility for the case. He has to do certain things on the night of admission to get the wheels turning: he must get an initial history from the patient and family, as well as write orders for the patient; he must formulate an initial therapeutic approach to the patient's illness and discuss this with the nurse on duty. Because he has begun treatment and may have already formed a good working relationship with the patient, it may be a disadvantage to change doctors, even if you do discover later that a more competent psychiatrist is available.

If, say, Dr. X is treating the patient and you find out that Dr. Y is the one you would rather have, I would suggest that you call Dr. Y or, even better, speak to him in person. Tell him, "Look, Uncle Filbert was hospitalized last night because we were afraid he was going to kill himself. Dr. X was on call and has started treatment, but he is not the doctor we would have chosen if we had had time to look into it. We would like to have you take the case but realize there are certain possible complications involved in switching. What is your feeling about this sort of thing?" Dr. Y may respond in a number of ways. Since he is a competent psychiatrist, he may realize that it would not be wise to tamper with the relationship that Uncle Filbert has already formed with Dr. X and, therefore, refuse to become involved. Or, his relationship with Dr. X may be good enough itself that they interchange patients occasionally and can work something out in this case—after discussing it with the patient. Or, once you have given him an idea of the problem, he too, may feel that Dr. X is not competent to handle it and take over the case at your request and with the patient's concurrence.

This last alternative takes a gutsy psychiatrist. He is going to have to go to Dr. X and say, "Uncle Filbert's family wants me to see him. Is it okay with you if I take over?" If he doesn't have a good working relationship with Dr. X, or if Dr. X has any hang-ups at all, that's war, man, and Dr. X is going to become immediately defensive and answer, "Well, what's wrong? He's already getting better. We put out the fire, and now we're working on this or that, and what's it to you anyway? Why waste all the time I've already put on the case?" That's another reason why Dr. Y will be reluctant to just take over. If he does decide to accept the case, he can argue further with Dr. X. "Well, how will you deal with his family now that you know they're not going to be happy seeing you? Treating the family is just as important as treating the patient, because he is going to have to go back and live with them eventually." There are pros and cons to both sides and, hopefully, the doctors will be mature enough to work it out with the patient's best interests in mind—but don't bet on it. If the hassle becomes too sticky, just accept the situation and stay with Dr. Y.

Members of the medical profession are prima donnas, and many find it difficult to accept a patient's switching doctors. Some are so sensitive that they actually become paranoid about it. They interpret it as a personal and professional rejection, an insult to their integrity, an accusation implying they had committed a crime. Doctors need to be brought down to earth. They are not heavenly beings who are perfect and, even if they were, the public still has a right to pick and choose among them and to change doctors when it seems advisable.

In my own city, there's an unwritten code among the physicians that one won't take over a case until the former doctor has released the patient. When I first ran into the code, I couldn't believe it! What the hell right does a doctor have to release his patients? Does he own them? I never "release" patients. They're free to come and go as they please, and I tell them so. Once a patient senses that his doctor feels threatened by rejection, or is on the defensive and hanging onto him like a personal possession, more psychological problems have been created than can possibly be solved—and, man that's bad medical practice, not only in psychiatry, but in other specialties as well. There's that gentleman's agreement— we won't slit each other's throats or grab patients out of each other's laps—not that it has anything to do with the best interest of the patients.

Competent physicians, including competent psychiatrists, will have their patients' well-being foremost in mind. That is why it is so important for you, the layman, to understand just what is going on behind the carefully rendered, sterile facades of the medical profession and to demand quality practice and services. That is why it is so essential for you to seek and find a competent psychiatrist, one who can steer you back to good mental health as quickly and as completely as possible.

FIRST IMPRESSIONS COUNT

Having selected a psychiatrist, you are now ready to begin. The next thing you have to do is set an appointment. Don't just call the office and expect a secretary to fix you up with an appointment next Friday at 2:30 P.M. In the first place, this particular psychiatrist may not even have a secretary. He may use an answering service to take his calls and return them later at his own convenience. Second, psychiatrists generally book their appointments in advance, so you should be prepared to work out a mutually convenient time. In this respect, it is no different from making an appointment with any other kind of doctor.

If the shrink does not have a secretary, and if you have left a message, how long do you wait for him to return the call? In my opinion, if you have to wait more than twenty-four hours (excluding weekends), the chances are that this particular man is not for you. He does not have a well-organized communication system. If you feel kindhearted, you might give him one more chance. Call again and wait twenty-four more hours. That's long enough—no matter how good the guy is supposed to be. He may be too busy to take your case, but he's certainly not too busy to return your call.

If he does not have a secretary, there is reason to be suspicious. He probably runs a very controlled kind of practice; his patients have to conform pretty well to his expectations. There is little opportunity for the kind of give-and-take that I feel is so important in a truly therapeutic doctor-patient relationship. The secretary is, in a sense, an extension of the doctor himself, and most people appreciate knowing that if some kind of emergency should arise, they will be able to call and, at least, talk to the secretary if the doctor is tied up or out of town on a particular day. So, if this is important to you, you had better think twice about the matter.

The secretary-receptionist is the psychiatrist's public relations department; you can reasonably expect her to be both courteous and efficient. She should have the authority to book your appointment. Her demeanor should boost the confidence you are beginning to build in the psychiatrist whom you have not yet seen. After all, he has hired this girl, and if he is not a good judge of her functional capacity to relate to his patients, there is reason to question his ability to evaluate your own functional capacity. Let the secretary be a tip-off to you in this respect. If the doctor relies primarily on some kind of automated recording device, I strongly urge you to look up another guy. You want human contact—and you want it even when calling for your appointment.

I am told that may psychiatrists will keep a prospective patient waiting several weeks before the initial appointment. If such is the case, you may safely conclude that he is too unresponsive to the immediate needs of his patients. Waste no time! Get yourself another boy! Generally speaking, a week to ten days is ample time to wait for your first appointment. A well-organized psychiatrist will purposely keep a flexible schedule so that he can accommodate new patients within that general time period.

The time has finally arrived for your first appointment! Most psychiatrists will be on time, give or take a few minutes. If you are late, do not expect him to prolong the hour beyond the appointed time. He probably has another patient to be seen then. So be on time—and, if he is late, let him know how you feel about it. I remember seeing a young college student recently. I was about twenty minutes behind schedule, and when she finally got to see me, she was so angry, she was unable to discuss her problems at all. When I pointed out to her that I was sorry that she had to wait so long, she managed to blurt out just how angry she was. As a result of this, her treatment became much more meaningful; she was able to lay her feelings more on the line, and her improvement was more rapid because of it. Psychiatrists do not as a rule purposely attempt to provoke anger; frustrating situations do arise, however, just as in real life and can't always be prevented.

Your first appointment will generally set the tone for all future ones. Go in prepared. You know he's going to ask you what your main problem is. Don't respond as do some patients I know: "Well, if I knew that, doctor, I wouldn't be here, would I?" He simply wants to know what led to your decision to come to see him. Another favorite gambit of the resistant patient is that he came because someone told him to come. This kind of evasiveness, if persistent, indicates that the person may not really want help; he is only trying to pacify the referring agent. Don't waste your time or the psychiatrist's playing such games. It is your job as a patient to size up the psychiatrist—as much or even more than it is his job to size you up. Reassure yourself in every way possible that this guy is competent, that he does not appear to be in need of help himself, and that he is the kind of guy you can confide in if given enough time to establish a comfortable working relationship.

In my own experience I have found that patients vary greatly in regard to establishing the working relationship. While some patients quickly establish a positive, confiding, and trustful relationship, others do not progress beyond a constantly mistrustful, suspicious, secretive kind of involvement that usually indicates a paranoid relation to all other people. Generally speaking, try to wait until two or three sessions have elapsed before you finally decide whether this is the guy for you. Unless, that is, it is very apparent to you in the very first session that he cannot possibly be of any real help to you.

Some of the observations that may lead you to a very rapid conclusion in this respect are as follows: he seems to take no personal interest in your case; he seems cold and overly analytic; he appears to be probing the depths of your mind without giving you the opportunity to get comfortable in your relationship with him; you get the feeling somehow that he is more interested in your unconscious than he is in you as a person; he makes you nervous, and therfore tends to turn you off rather than on. If such is the case, call in before your next appointment and cancel out.

A quick negative decision is also warranted if the psychiatrist is too quick to talk about himself and his own problems. Such psychiatrists will frequently have pictures of their wives and children in the office. This may become very distracting and prevent you from focusing on your own problems—reasons why you came to see him in the first place. After all, you are paying him—not vice versa. Also, you do not go to a psychiatrist to have lengthy discussions about the world situation or who the best candidate for public office may be. Above all, you want a psychiatrist who sticks to the problem at hand. Don't settle for less.

Another quick turn-off that a lot of shrinks pull is to waste the entire first hour asking a lot of irrelevant questions about your past life. Without any real sense of direction, they wander from question to question, asking first about your symptoms, then about your mother and father, then your sex life, and finally about your oldest sister's third marriage. This guy is filling up the hour with irrelevant questions because he never learned how to get a proper psychiatric history. Get rid of him even though you may enjoy the attention for its own sake. He doesn't know where he's going with all these questions—and if he doesn't know, how the hell are you going to figure it out?

Equally if not more frustrating is the guy who never gives you a direct answer to any of the questions you ask. When asked by a very depressed patient if she is going to get better, he responds, "Your guess is as good as mine," or "That depends on a large number of variables over which I have no control." Don't put up with that kind of horse manure. You want someone who talks straight to you. Otherwise, you are never going to learn how to talk straight to him. Tell the guy you have had it and go find yourself a more qualified psychiatrist.

After all, the true art and science of psychiatry consists basically in the psychiatrist's capacity to initiate, sustain, and resolve a meaningful dialogue between himself and the patient, a dialogue that will significantly undermine the roots of the patient's illness. The start of that dialogue occurs the moment you enter that office. If you are human you don't want to waste time getting the job done. Don't pussyfoot around with the bastard if he's not on the ball. So far, you have only invested the cost of one hour—not ten, twenty, fifty, or a hundred. God knows how many people have spent untold thousands on headshrinkers who were competent only in sending out their monthly bills. Your first contact with the psychiatrist should provide you with very distinct impressions regarding the correctness of your choice. Pay attention to your feelings and check them out over the next few sessions. The kind of relationship that develops between you and him will determine the success or failure of the whole operation.

CHAPTER **5**

Ask And Ye Shall Receive

"THE TRUE ART and science of psychiatry lies
basically in the psychiatrist's capacity to initiate, sustain,
and resolve a meaningful dialogue between himself and
the patient, one that will significantly undermine the
roots of the patient's illness." If only someone had told
me that during my first, second, or even third year of
residency training. I think I could have become a more
competent psychiatrist a lot sooner. As it was, I did not
really begin to appreciate the significance of the relationship between doctor and patient until I saw a skit put on
by the patients at McLean. To be sure, they were poking
fun at the psychiatrists, caricaturing the way each of us
appeared to them as we conducted our daily rounds.

As I recall, very few psychiatrists attended this performance; I know that I was apprehensive myself, waiting to see how the patients would portray me. They
characterized me as an absent-minded professor who had
trouble responding directly to even their simplest questions. Though it was difficult for me to join in with the
laughter of the patients, I knew immediately that they

were essentially correct in their appraisal of me. In retrospect, I was so concerned that I would put my foot in my mouth or say the wrong thing that I ended up by not saying very much at all in my relationship with patients. They felt cheated by me—and they were right. Most training programs overemphasize the therapist's need to be right at the expense of his need to be spontaneous. That skit, perhaps more than anything else, started me thinking about the psychiatrist-patient relationship as perceived by the patient. Previously, I had seen it only through the eyes of the psychiatrist. I was beginning to finally comprehend that this relationship is a two-way street, and the psychiatrist must be constantly aware of how he appears to the patient—not in the limited sense of transference—but as a total human being.

This is precisely why you will never be able to program a computer to do psychotherapy. Yet this kind of research goes on—in the name of science! People in the field of mental health who are so divorced from their own humanity that they prefer working with machines, especially computers, should stay in the laboratory working with rats. When they get a little better, they can graduate to monkeys and chimpanzees. Let them stay away from patients, however, at least until they have been in treatment themselves for a sufficiently long period of time to recognize the differences.

Bearing in mind the types of psychiatrist described in Chapter 2, their shortcomings can best be understood in the context of the relationship between the patient and his psychiatrist. The Imitation Analyst does not relate to his patient as a unique human being. He hears only what he wants to hear. Hiding behind his intellectual theories, he protects himself from the unexpected. He's afraid to meet the patient head-on and so he sidesteps the relationship. From his side of the relationship, the patient either plays these petty intellectual games or, if he's smart, drops out of treatment. Such a relationship is too sterile to produce the kind of emotional insight that promotes healthy psychological change.

The Doktor is too busy playing doctor to tune in on the right wave length. He keeps the patient a long arms-reach away and hides behind his authoritarian front. The patient either knuckles under because of his own insecurity or he recognizes, finally, that he is being had. The Pigeon-Holer uses his labels to put the patient down. In this way he dehumanizes the relationship. It takes a very masochistic person to tolerate this kind of treatment. The Swinger avoids genuine human contact by experimenting with his subjects. The patient is merely a guinea pig to him. An authentic relationship cannot take place. The Organization Man hooks his patient into the system, attempting thereby to get him off his back. Let the therapeutic mill grind out another product, regardless of the quality of service rendered. He depersonalizes the relationship and thus dooms it to failure. Our Problem Shrink distorts the relationship due to his inability to be objective. The patient is perceived merely as an extension of his own problems. Good Joe regards each new patient as a lifelong buddy who will share with him the loneliness of old age.

It should be apparent by now that anyone seeking to get his money's worth out of psychiatry must know something about the process of psychotherapy. He must know what the various stages of treatment are and how to detect whether or not the treatment is progressing from one stage to another in an orderly fashion. Only then will he know how to speed things up, what questions to ask, and how to evaluate the answers. Only then will he be able to determine whether the answers really make sense or merely create impediments to the development of a therapeutic-psychiatrist relationship. He must learn to ask the right questions if he is to receive the proper responses. This relationship depends as much on the patient as it does on the shrink. Two losers can't make a winner. When it comes to this business of psychotherapy, you want to do everything in your power to make it a winner. To do so, you must invest yourself as well as your money; by doing so, you may even be able to compensate for some of the inadequacies of your psychiatrist. After all, even the competent ones are human, and they too, occasionally goof.

THE STAGES OF THERAPY

There is an interesting paradox inherent in the psychiatrist-patient relationship. In one sense, it is a completely unreal situation. You go into this guy's office once or twice a week, whatever the case may be, and you tell him all about yourself, trying not to withhold anything that may be important. You expose yourself psychologically, in a way that is not feasible in a real life situation. You literally pour your guts out to the guy sitting across from you. You talk about all those feelings that are generally considered taboo—rage, shame, jealousy, and guilt. You talk to him, as though he were a long lost friend, and only occasionally does he talk back. When he does, it is basically to help you, the patient. This relationship is unreal because it cannot be transposed onto other relationships in real life. There is no other situation that's exactly equivalent to it in terms of the degree of intimacy, confidentiality, mutual respect, and objectivity.

On the other hand, because of the depth of the relationship and the kinds of feelings that can and must be expressed, there is a sense in which this relationship is more real than any other. At its best, it becomes a true vitalizing force that enriches a person's life far beyond any other interpersonal experience. (In this sense, anyone who wants to can benefit from psychotherapy.) It's because the relationship is so very profound that it is paradoxically both real and unreal—like good drama, in the sense that the characters in the play use, as their taking off point, real life situations, but the dramatic intensity is so great that it transcends life itself. I suppose you could say there is a sort of religious quality, but more importantly, an aesthetic depth to the psychiatrist-patient relationship that does not pertain to the kinds of relationships that a person has with other people—any other people.

Like any other relationship, however, it too can go wrong at various points. The alert person can prevent this from happening if he is aware of some of the basic pitfalls that can occur. Even at best, of course, the relationship does not go perfectly smoothly.

There are four phases in the development of this relationship. The first, or testing phase, is characterized by the initial tendency of a patient to test out the relationship in terms of how far he can go with the psychiatrist, how much he should expose himself, and whether he can trust this guy who sets himself up as a healer of the mind. He needs to prove to his own satisfaction that going to a headshrinker was really a good idea in the first place.

Patients vary considerably in how long they stay in phase one. I remember one gal who was quite paranoid and never really got beyond this stage. She was constantly challenging me, making such remarks as, "I don't agree with that" or "That isn't true," "How do you know that for sure?" everytime I opened my mouth, no matter how benevolent I tried to be. With this type of patient, of course, the problem of trust is foremost. They aren't able to trust anyone and the psychiatrist really has to work hard in order to get the relationship going. To a certain extent, all patients withhold their trust in this initial phase of treatment. It is natural—and wise—for them to do so. The paranoid patient sometimes can't get beyond this point because, previously, everyone he had ever trusted betrayed him. The build-up of feelings of suspicion and mistrust is so great that even the competent psychiatrist must strain considerably in order to penetrate the initial barrier. I certainly don't recommend, however, that you go in with complete trust and admiration for a headshrinker when you know nothing about him except that somebody has recommended him, even though that recommendation may have been very complimentary. You still need to establish your own personal working relationship with this guy. Don't sell yourself short by immediately putting him up on a tremendous pedestal that he may not deserve.

There are, of course, some patients who come into the office and are very trusting right from the start. They seem to feel that the psychiatrist can do no wrong. This naïvete is usually connected with their reasons for seeing a psychiatrist in the first place. A very common instance of this is the young adult female who immediately trusts any man who even appears to be concerned about her welfare. She usually finds herself deeply involved with a series of men, each affair ending in complete rejection by the man, much to her chagrin and disappointment. She has no concept of why "fate" has treated her so unkindly. I have to teach such a patient to be less trusting and a little more suspicious of members of the opposite sex.

During this testing phase, a male patient frequently, in a symbolic way, compares the size of his penis with that of the psychiatrist. One patient currently in treatment makes statements like: "Why should I have to come to you; you're just a human being like I am; I'm just as smart as you are; I've built up a big business on my own hook, why should I need you?" This kind of preoccupation represents not only a lack of trust but also a fear of dependence on the therapist. He needs to test the therapist out in terms of whether or not he will be rejected (as he probably was by his father).

After the testing phase, many patients resort to a stage of complete compliance. During this state of dependence, they are very humble and subservient to the therapist. They will do almost anything to please him. Some will even try to be entertaining by telling him the latest jokes they have heard. They are very submissive and hang on his every word. Overly dependent on the therapist now that he has passed their tests, they feel that they can let it all hang out and put themselves completely at his disposal.

In a sense, this behavior has some merit because it means that the patient finally does trust the therapist and is now prepared to disclose some of the underlying conflicts and feelings in a way that may be productive. The main danger, however, is that the patient will in fact become overly dependent on the psychiatrist and overly sensitive to rejection or what he is apt to interpret as rejection. One patient recently chastised me for not having noticed that she was wearing her hair differently. Another obviously felt slighted when he reported to me that he had changed his job to a much more lucrative and prestigious one, and I didn't appear to be terribly impressed by this revelation.

It is during the dependency phase of therapy that the competent psychiatrist really stands out from all the other types. He is able to handle the nuances in the relationship with such skill, both verbal and nonverbal, that the patient is able to work through his feelings toward the therapist at the very time he is beginning to resolve his underlying problems. This is accomplished by connecting the patient's feelings about the therapist with the conflicts he is having in relation to the important people in his life. The therapist helps the patient to integrate things in such a way that he can then see a pattern underlying his emotional reactions. By so doing, the excessive dependency is diluted down to workable proportions.

For example, the man who felt the therapist was not praising him sufficiently for the positive action he had taken in changing jobs, expressed it through his feeling that his wife did not sufficiently appreciate him. I immediately asked him why he expected her to be so appreciative when he was merely doing what he should have done a long time ago. In asking him this question, I not only got his wife off the hook, so to speak, but also got myself out of potential trouble by focusing the problem back on him and the origins of his feeling that other people do not sufficiently appreciate him. This feeling could then be traced back to his relationship with his parents, where it rightfully belonged. In other words, the therapist must be keenly alert to the cues from his patient and be ready to exploit them fully as the need arises.

If during this phase a patient finds himself constantly scolding or criticizing the therapist for one reason or another (it makes no difference if those reasons are imaginary or real), it may well be that the therapist is not doing his job adequately. In other words, he is not helping the patient trace in sufficient historical perspective the real roots of his neurotic feelings. He simply is not in tune with what's going on.

It should be fairly clear by now that the therapist, though a very real person, is only a catalyst in the sense that he helps the patient to trace back the sources of his anxieties and conflicts so that he can work out the basis for them. The woman who felt resentful because I had not noticed her new hairdo was merely projecting her anger toward her husband, who generally paid little or no attention to her personal appearance. It was not difficult to place this feeling where it rightfully belonged, and I did so immediately. Not to have done so would have led to the possible build up of feelings of resentment projected onto the therapist from other sources. The positive relationship must be preserved sufficiently to maintain the patient's trust and confidence.

The competent psychiatrist, therefore, walks a very fine line between encouraging too much dependency, love, or devotion and too much resentment, feeling of rejection, or anger. I say it's a very fine line because that's exactly what it is. How fine a line depends, of course, on the degree of the patient's psychopathology and how disturbed he was to start with. In its most extreme form, a patient will one day want to murder the psychiatrist and the next, to worship him. Working through these ambivalent feelings to their logical conclusion, by examining the way in which they developed, is the psychiatrist's main job. To the extent that he is successful in this effort—to that extent and only to that extent—will the patient get over his basic hang-ups.

The third phase of therapy refers to the time during the treatment when the patient can relate to the psychiatrist fairly objectively, as just another human being who happens to have a certain expertise in helping people to better understand themselves. During this objective phase of treatment, the relationship is basically a healthy one. There is no further testing to be done nor is there any tendency to be overly compliant with the therapist. Further, the patient is not easily slighted by anything the therapist might say or do. The therapy can progress, no longer obstructed by the patient's tendencies to project onto the psychiatrist any magical powers or similar infantile feelings. During this phase of treatment, the work that has to be done proceeds relatively smoothly. By this stage, the patient has learned how to relate to the psychiatrist without expecting too much or receiving too little. He knows where it's at, so to speak, and it usually isn't long after this phase has started that he begins dropping some clues that he is ready to try it on his own. The patient himself makes the decision regarding when the treatment is over.

He is now ready to enter the final phase, the stage of independence from the therapist. Treatment is terminated by mutual consent of patient and psychiatrist. Both parties know that he does not have to come in anymore. The therapy goes on even after the actual sessions have terminated. Assuming the therapy has been successful, a patient will recall frequently, as new situations arise that would previously have led to symptoms, how the doctor would have responded to the situation. It is not unusual for a patient to carry on an imaginary conversation with the therapist a long time after having discontinued treatment. The more successful it has been, the more successful such imaginary sessions are in resolving the new difficulties. This does not mean that patients are not invited to come back for a session or two if the need should arise in the future. Frequently they will need to return to discuss the new developments in person, but such sessions are usually few in number and can be spaced at progressively longer intervals.

By separating out these four different stages of therapy in terms of the relationship between psychiatrist and patient, I do not mean that one stage follows the other always either chronologically or in pure form. In each phase there are elements of the other three. The treatment does, however, follow this general pattern.

EVALUATING THE TREATMENT

Are there ways that a patient can surmise whether or not his treatment is progressing in a satisfactory fashion? Many shrinks would violently oppose the idea that the patient is in as good a position to evaluate the course of his treatment as the psychiatrist himself. I am not referring now to the acutely disturbed or psychotic patient, but I am referring to all the rest. Psychiatrists have for too long put themselves in the position of being beyond questioning. Yet there are some rather obvious criteria that may be used by most patients to determine if they are truly getting their money's worth. The following principles are stated not so much in their order of importance as in logical sequence. They are questions that any patient may ask at any time in the course of his therapy.

1. *"Does the psychiatrist appear to be genuinely concerned and interested in me?"* Different shrinks reflect concern with their patients in different ways. That they must indicate this concern and make it clearly evident to the patient, especially during the testing phase of therapy, may appear too obvious to mention. Yet I can assure you that it is violated repeatedly by headshrinkers who, in their phony attempts to be scientific, are themselves relatively oblivious to the human factors involved. You have every reason in the world to expect psychiatrists to show a deep concern about your health and welfare from the psychological point of view. If you don't get it to the degree that you feel you need it, the sooner you tell him

that he seems too cold and unfeeling to meet your needs, the sooner you will resolve a serious obstacle to the progress in the treatment.

2. *"Is the psychiatrist so concerned, however, that he is not really in control of the treatment?"* No matter how experienced the psychiatrist may be, there are instances when he will tend to overidentify with the patient and his problems. The psychiatrist must, at all times, be in control of the treatment process in the sense of providing a certain degree of leadership. I don't mean the kind of leadership demonstrated by a benevolent dictator. I do mean the kind of leadership that provides a model of maturity in terms of the kinds of conflicts that the patient brings into the office. The therapist must be a constant reminder of the ways in which the disturbed person is contributing to his own dilemma. There is no room for pussyfooting around in this respect. Another way of asking this question is whether or not the sessions with the psychiatrist are really any different from bull sessions that one might have with a friend.

One of the most disturbing things to me about the quality of psychiatric practice today is the "conspiracy of nondirection." This conspiracy is based on the kind of relationship that frequently develops between a psychiatrist and his patient wherein the psychiatrist ends up doing nothing, more or less, than supporting the patient's inadequacies in a way that merely tends to perpetuate the underlying conflicts and problems. Nothing ever really happens. The treatment remains fixated at phase two, the stage of dependency—and it never gets beyond that point. This kind of conspiracy is most common in the practices of those shrinks who cater to the carriage trade. The rich, neurotic patient keeps coming back with the same old dreary complaints, and the shrink merely maintains a facade of sympathy and concern without ever coming to grips with the basic issues involved. How desperate can a person be to make a living?

The conspiracy of nondirection received considerable impetus from the fact that for such a long time psychiatrists have been taught to use a basically nondirective technique. A nondirective technique is simply one where the patient is given complete freedom to provide the direction of the therapy, and the psychiatrist merely tends to repeat the last word or ask for clarification in some other way. The shrink, remaining basically passive in this procedure, hopes somehow that the patient will then go ahead and spell out all of the problems in such a way that he will automatically get better. This is the technique that has been satirized so frequently by such jokes as the patient telling the psychiatrist that he is now planning to jump out the window and the psychiatrist responding with, "The window?" whereupon the patient promptly does a swan dive to the pavement below.

I would say, unequivocally, that there can be no such thing as a completely nondirective technique. It means only a *lack* of direction in the treatment, and treatment that has no direction is doomed to failure. Unfortunately, some patients get so much enjoyment out of such a conspiracy with the shrink that they will keep coming back for the rest of their lives. Whoever said that you had to be rich in order to qualify for good medical treatment in this country certainly didn't have psychiatry in mind when he made the statement. Good Joe, of course, loves to be nondirective. Using this technique, he can always blame the patient for not getting well.

3. *"Does he understand me?"* Having established the fact that the psychiatrist is concerned about you and, further, that he is in control of the treatment, you must then ask yourself if he really understands you. Never assume that he does. As a matter of fact, the competent

psychiatrist frequently responds to his patient's statements with, "I don't understand, what do you mean by
that?" He forces the patient to clarify and explain exactly what he means, over and over again, until the underlying roots of the problem become apparent. There is
really one way, therefore, to tell whether the psychiatrist
understands you and that is by determining if he helps
you to understand yourself. If he only appears to be understanding, the chances are that he doesn't understand at
all. You need to have definite feedback, indicating clearly
that he understands exactly how you feel and the nature
of your problems. If you don't get this kind of feedback,
you have reason to be suspicious of him and his capacity
to treat you.

The long history-taking type of psychiatrist, who
seems to be asking questions for their own sake apart
from any direct relevance to your problems, is the worst
culprit in this respect. He goes off in all directions looking for something that may strike his fancy. Even if
he does stumble accidently upon an area of conflict, there
is no assurance that resolving that area will help the
patient with the particular problems that led to his seeking help in the first place. Make no mistake about the fact
that everything a psychiatrist says and does during the
treatment has to have a damn good reason.

4. *"Do I understand him?"* This is perhaps the most
basic question of all, for the answer to it determines
whether the psychiatrist is capable of communicating
adequately with you, the patient, about the things that
matter most. You may be fascinated by his intellectual
prowess and psychological insights, you may be en-
thralled by his command of the English language, your
gonads may twitch every time he opens his mouth, but
the question remains and has to be answered: Do you
really understand what the hell this guy is communicating

to you and understand it on a gut level where it really counts?

The psychiatrist's ability to communicate with any given patient depends on many variables, not the least of which are his inborn talent and the quality of his training. The acid test of his worth to you is how well he communicates with you on a level that you can understand. After all, it is largely on the basis of this newly acquired understanding that you must begin to rearrange your attitudes and behavior.

One very common way in which psychiatrists fail to communicate adequately is the way in which they slough off some of the questions that patients ask. Any question not only deserves to be answered but deserves to be answered in a way that the patient can clearly understand. The shrink's right to ask you questions is no more sacred than your right to ask questions of him. Assuming, of course, that you are doing your best to answer his questions, then he must do no less for you. How many times have I heard patients complain that they never knew what the doctor was thinking. How many times have I heard these same patients tell me that their former shrinks never would answer their questions. There are times when I feel I should go to the next meeting of the American Psychiatric Association and pass out a little card to every member in attendance, and on that card would be written in boldface type the simple statement: *PATIENTS ARE HUMAN—TREAT THEM WITH RESPECT—GIVE THEM DIRECT ANSWERS TO THEIR QUESTIONS.*

Another indication of whether the communication is taking place as it should is the presence or absence of a mutual understanding between patient and psychiatrist regarding the exact goals of the treatment. I am convinced that a large number of patients keep going back without having the foggiest notion of the goals of the treatment. I know this must be true because the psychiatrist himself in so many instances has no clear idea. So, if you have reason to suspect that the psychiatrist is not really on target, that he is not communicating on your wave length, one way of checking is to ask him directly about the goals of the treatment. If the answer does not satisfy you fully, keep working on him until he comes up with a reasonable explanation. Hopefully, you will be able to resolve it in short order; if not, you have every reason to doubt that you are getting your money's worth.

If all four of these questions are answered affirmatively, you may feel relatively sure that you are on the road to recovery. If the kind of communication that I have described is in fact taking place, you will feel free enough and secure enough in the relationship to gradually expose your underlying conflicts, and the psychiatrist will be able to help you resolve them. You will begin to feel better and more confident, your symptoms will tend to disappear gradually, and you will experience a sense of liberation. In short, as time goes on, you will know that you are getting better: you will be able to do things that you could not do before; you'll make decisions that before seemed impossible; you'll resolve problems that previously seemed insurmountable; you will not merely be better adjusted, you will be a more complete and fulfilled human being. Don't settle for any less than this; you owe it to yourself, and the psychiatrist owes it to you—assuming you pay your bill, that is.

5. *"Is this guy's technique generally consistent with accepted standards of psychiatric treatment?"* There are so many weird varieties of psychotherapy around today that it behooves the patient to inquire if his psychiatrist is using techniques that are generally accepted by the profession. Despite what I may have implied earlier,

there is at least one principle of technique that has stood
the test of time and is necessarily part of any competent
therapist's armamentarium—the general principle of
relating current problems to past conflicts. This need to
relate present and past patterns of feeling and behavior
is an essential ingredient of any psychiatrist's technique.
It's not enough just to ventilate feelings; it's not enough
simply to talk about one's early childhood; it's not enough
merely to understand the build-up of intense feeling during one's early life. The single most important principle
of psychiatric technique is the capacity to relate present
problems to the development of conflicts in one's early
life.

Any psychiatrist who deviates radically from this
technique is open to the accusation that he is trying to
develop a unique style of treatment at the expense of the
accumulated experience of all the competent psychiatrists who have preceded him. No matter how novel the
technique, no matter how much it turns you on, and no
matter what the apparent results, I would think twice
about continuing treatment with a psychiatrist who does
not attempt in some fashion to correlate present and past.
Understanding the present can only be accomplished
through understanding the past and vice versa.

Don't get confused about this. The Imitation Analyst,
for example, will keep you talking about the past so much
that you may temporarily forget about the problems
you're having in the present. Overemphasizing the former
at the expense of the latter is just as wrong as the technique that emphasizes the present at the expense of the
past. There is one other aspect of technique, although it
does not apply to all patients, that is, the need of the
psychiatrist, at times, to offer specific guidance or techniques that a patient may use in dealing with his individual symptoms. A certain percentage of patients are

so up tight about their phobias or interpersonal problems that it behooves the psychiatrist to give them some tips on how to cope with the situation. These tips are not merely gimmicks nor do they constitute the essence of the treatment. They must be designed specifically to give the patient something concrete to work with. Something he can hold onto in order to avoid the panicky feeling of which many patients complain so bitterly.

I'm not talking here about oversimplified techniques such as "the power of positive thinking." I am talking about some of the techniques used by Recovery, Inc. The simple statement, for example, that the patient's symptoms are "distressing but not dangerous" is frequently very helpful to the anxious patient. These techniques serve a very useful purpose if they help the patient to consciously control his overwhelming feelings of anxiety so that he can better focus on the underlying problems. Though frowned upon by traditional psychoanalysts and by so-called "non-directive" therapists, such strategy is an essential ingredient in the treatment of many emotionally disturbed people. If you have reason to believe the shrink just leaves you hanging in outer space, that he is not providing you with any solid foundation on which to stand, discuss this with him. The longer you go on dangling from his pedestal, the greater your chances of falling from it.

These are your guidelines. Use them. Assert yourself when the need arises. Only by doing so will you get your money's worth. Keep pressing until you are satisfied on all five of the principles.

HOW TO GET BETTER RESULTS IN LESS TIME

Bearing in mind the four stages of therapy and the five guidelines for evaluating the quality of treatment, what can the average person do to minimize results and minimize the time involved? First of all, remember that it is never too late to switch therapists if you are dissatisfied with the way things are going. You must, however, have good reasons to do so. One valid reason would be the fact that your shrink, despite the fact that you followed the selection process outlined in Chapter 4, turned out to be one of the incompetent types described in Chapter 2, e.g., an Imitation Analyst or Doktor or Swinger, etc. Simply recognize the fact that you made a mistake and begin again with someone else.

Assuming that you have been fortunate enough to find a competent psychiatrist, what can you do to speed things up and to get the most out of treatment. Just as there are five ways to evaluate the treatment or relationship between yourself and the therapist, there are five corresponding methods that you can use to move things along to their natural conclusion.

1. If for any reason and at any time, you feel that the psychiatrist is not showing sufficient concern for you or some aspect of your problem, let him know about it right away. Don't pass this feeling off as childish or irrelevant. What will happen if you are too shy or too embarrassed to discuss it with him? You will not only increase your defensive resistance to therapy but will also miss one of the best opportunities to really get at the heart of things. The competent psychiatrist loves this kind of self-expression because it invariably leads to the gradual unfolding of many, if not all, of a patient's underlying conflicts. This is no time for pussyfooting around. Let it all hang out, but be prepared to trace the conflicts back to their childhood precursors because that is exactly what you are paying this guy to help you do. Don't make a federal case out of it. Just get it off your chest and begin working it out with the doctor's help.

2. If it appears that the shrink is not exercising sufficient control or direction over the course of treatment,
discuss this with him. After all, this is exactly what you
are paying him for. He expresses his knowledge and skill
in the way he guides the conversation and facilitates your
treatment. If he appears to be slacking in some way, or
not providing you with the kind of leadership that you
feel necessary, let him know the specifics of how you feel
and why. It can only help matters; it can't hurt. Many
patients are so fearful of hurting people's feelings that it
takes them forever even to tell their psychiatrist what it
is about him that they don't like! The longer you give
into this specific fear as it relates to the psychiatrist himself, the bigger your bill will be. Loosen up and tell him
what you think because if you don't, he'll never know.
You are the one who has to pay the bill each month, not
him.

This whole business of learning how to express one's
feelings about other people is the crux of all psychotherapy. First, to be able to express the feelings and then,
to understand how and why. The expression is more
important than the how and why, though both are necessary. Feelings about oneself and one's own body are
just as important as feelings toward other people. So
come into those sessions prepared to emote. Don't just
sit back and use the hour as a break from your usual routine. If that's all you want, go and have a cup of coffee
with your neighbors or a drink with the boys. Don't waste
your time and money on psychotherapy. It's not for you.

3. If at any time the shrink doesn't seem to understand what you're trying to tell him (believe me, this
does happen frequently), stop right there and spell it out
more clearly until it begins to penetrate. I am always asking patients what they mean when they say something
that isn't crystal clear. The psychiatrist *must* understand.

If he indicates that he misinterpreted something you said or a feeling that you expressed, lay it on him again. If you fail to do so, the communication will bog down and so will the treatment. More time will be required and your pocketbook will get lighter. This should not happen too often if the psychiatrist is really qualified, but it does happen often enough for you to bear it in mind. If it occurs repeatedly, you have reason to question whether you made the right choice. This is another valid indication for switching therapists.

4. When the psychiatrist makes a statement that you do not fully and immediately comprehend, ask him to explain it as many times as necessary. Don't blithely continue your discussion of other matters. After all, you're paying for those words of wisdom. Therapy is a dialogue, not a soliloquy. You may enjoy hearing yourself talk, but you are in that office to communicate, not to stage a one-man show. Also, don't be afraid the shrink will think you are stupid if you ask him what he means. He will interpret the question as a sign of intelligence on your part because it demonstrates the fact that you recognize the importance of understanding what he says. He will also know that you are serious about wanting to get over whatever it is that's bugging you.

I cannot emphasize too strongly how important this is—assuming, of course, that you want to make rapid progress. So many patients don't even hear the therapist for a long time. I frequently find myself having to interrupt the session rather abruptly, do something to make sure I have the person's full attention and then hammer the point home as if I were talking to someone who was partially deaf. I find this an extremely useful technique but one that I wish I did not have to use so often. You really do need an experienced psychiatrist since it is unlikely that any novice in the field can assert himself that forcefully.

If the shrink frequently makes statements that are incomprehensible to you, chances are he is not able to communicate on your wave length. This is a bad sign. Don't ignore it for too long. If things don't improve rapidly, cancel out and look elsewhere. Too many shrinks still talk a lot of technical mumbo jumbo. Their jargon only confuses instead of enlightens the patient. Since he is pretty confused to start with, the situation can only deteriorate further.

5. Pay attention to whether or not you are concentrating exclusively on current events or past experiences. Some patients will come in and concentrate only on their present hang-ups. It's like pulling teeth sometimes to get them off one subject and onto another—like the hypochondriac who can discuss only the aches and pains of the day. Try to keep the conversation flowing from one area to another and from one time period to another. Your therapist will aid you in this task, but you can help by not getting fixated on one special topic. There are times when the psychiatrist will choose to focus on one special area but, generally speaking, things need to flow back and forth from one sector to another though they may all be linked together in some way. As a matter of fact, that is how a person develops insight into his problems, by seeing connections between things and events that appeared initially to be entirely unrelated.

If you have any questions about any technique the shrink uses, ask him for clarification. Expect him to challenge you fairly directly if you tell him that you *can't* do something that you obviously must do in order to get well. I frequently tell patients that the word "can't" does not exist in my vocabulary. They soon get the idea and stop making such remarks as, "I can't stand to be alone" or "I can't stop thinking this way." Soon they ask if I think they can get well, and the obvious answer is that I *know* they can, if they really want to. In other words, the psychiatrist must believe in you even if you don't believe in yourself. This is the test of both his concern about you and his control of the therapy. These issues must be resolved during the early testing phase of treatment. During the stage of dependence, however, is when you must pay the most attention to your feelings toward the psychiatrist, and he must be most keenly aware of his feelings toward you. Many a therapy has been botched up at this point, either because the patient was unable to tolerate the dependence, or the psychiatrist did not handle it skillfully. Avoid becoming excessively dependent on the therapist at this point. Avoid also becoming any more hostile toward him than the real situation warrants. Remember that your ambivalent feelings toward him have been conditioned by your experiences with other people—both past and present. Discuss your feelings with him. Don't take them out on him.

SOME PATIENTS ARE TOUGH

There are certain attitudes that some patients will project onto the psychiatrist that make treatment more difficult. The following descriptions of these patient types are intentionally exaggerated in order to highlight the ways in which they undermine their own treatment. Because of this, the stages of therapy are much more prolonged than they have to be, theoretically, and it is more difficult to evaluate the course of treatment at any given moment.

THE MIRACLE SEEKER

This patient has usually been struggling with severe problems for many years, then suddenly gets it into his head that he wants psychiatric treatment. He comes in expecting miracles, expecting the headshrinker to wave his magic wand and thus dispose of all the turmoil. He seems to equate going to a psychiatrist with having a surgical procedure performed that will instantly and dramatically remove all of his pathology. He becomes quite frustrated early in the therapy when he suddenly realizes that psychotherapy does not involve magic but actually requires a lot of hard work on the part of both the patient and the psychiatrist. The competent psychiatrist, of course, educates the patient about the process of psychotherapy. He tends to be rather tolerant of such an attitude because he knows how much the patient has been suffering. He points out to the patient, repeatedly, that psychiatry is not like surgery in this respect and that the patient himself must seek out and find his own answers. The therapist is simply a catalyst for helping the patient in this exploratory process. The Miracle Seeker is very naïve in this respect, tending to be overly dependent on the psychiatrist, as he has been on all other authority figures in his life. In seeking a miracle treatment he betrays his complete lack of confidence in his own capacity to work out problems even with the help of an expert.

THE BELLYACHER

This person sees the psychiatrist as someone to use as a wailing wall and nothing more. He comes in and recites his many complaints, which seem to be endless. One day it's a stomachache, the next day, a headache. Then it's how badly his children are behaving or that his wife is constantly putting him down. Whether or not he gets any relief from the mere recital, over and over again, of his many symptoms, he has considerable difficulty realizing that the purpose of seeing a psychiatrist is not merely to gripe and complain but to attempt the kind of self-understanding that will enable him to master the conflicts underlying his symptoms. The competent psychiatrist recognizes the patient's need to obtain some symptomatic relief and will probably prescribe some medication. However, the purpose in doing so is merely to encourage the patient to begin gradually to relate to him in a way that will lead to the resolution of his problems. The Bellyacher is frequently overwhelmed with self-pity and tends to see himself as the victim of circumstances over which he has no control. Like the Miracle Seeker, he tends to look for a supernatural cure rather than to face up to his real problems. Many psychiatrists tend to turn off such patients as not being fit candidates for psychotherapy. Though in some cases this may be true, I am frequently amazed to discover how, with a firm and consistent approach, one can help such patients begin to look at themselves more objectively and understand why it is that they have so many complaints. Once it finally begins to penetrate that they are not unique or so very different from other people, they are then able to settle down and begin figuring out why and how they happen to have so many gripes. The underlying frustrations begin to emerge, and they begin to understand why they chose this particular form of defense against their feelings.

THE SEDUCER

This is the type of female who has always related to men on the basis of her sexual charms. She can't resist the same temptation with the psychiatrist and tends to sexualize the relationship to the extent that it interferes with her treatment. The Seducer has frequently tried to dominate men through her provocative behavior and has usually ended up being rejected by them. The competent psychiatrist will, in most cases, recognize this in the very first interview. He will then structure the relationship quite clearly for the patient so that her conscious and unconscious fantasies don't get the better of her. As a first year resident, I remember being faked out by such a patient, as many first year residents are. The result was that she developed so positive an attraction to me that her sexual fantasies about me took the place of her entire neurotic illness. I was too inexperienced to cope with it adequately at the time, and all that my frustrated supervisor could say was that it was too late to do anything about it. Like anyone else I guess we shrinks sometimes have to learn the hard way. Needless to say, that was one patient who did not improve as a result of my efforts. If anything, she got worse.

THE MASOCHIST

This patient feels that he was born to suffer and actually appears to enjoy doing so. He relates to the psychiatrist as father confessor, and no amount of apparent forgiveness seems to assuage his guilty conscience. Whenever he begins to feel somewhat better, he finds ways and reasons again to make himself miserable. At these times, he wants the psychiatrist to rebuke him for his real and imagined transgressions. The competent psychiatrist really has his work cut out for him here. He must help the patient understand the repetitive nature of his guilt-atonement complex. The more masochistic the patient, the more difficult it is to accomplish this feat. Such patients require a very firm approach at times if they are to be made aware of just what they are doing to themselves and why—before they are able to change significantly. This self-destructive tendency, of course, reaches its most extreme form in the chronically suicidal patient.

THE HUNGRY MOUTH

This type of patient is fixated at a very infantile level of development. He comes into the office and throws himself at your mercy. He wants to be fed with all kinds of medication, advice, psychotherapy, and anything else that you can give him. The last thing he wants to do is assume any responsibility for his own behavior or make any real effort to understand himself. Such a person tries the patience of even the most competent psychiatrist. One has to spend many long hours with Hungry Mouth, helping him to understand even the basic fundamentals of what being a grown-up, mature person means. He resists you at every turn, expressing his helplessness to deal with even the simplest problems. The competent therapist must improvise a great deal with such a patient. He has every right to use unconventional techniques to stimulate him in a positive direction. Hungry Mouth taxes the ingenuity of a psychiatrist perhaps more than any other type of patient because most of the time he seems to be saying that he refuses to grow up. No one has the right, of course, to criticize the shrink unduly when this patient does not appear to be responding rapidly to treatment. The Good Joe psychiatrist will tend to become overly involved with such a patient in terms of trying to meet all of his infantile demands, and it is difficult to get past the first phase of therapy in such cases.

THE STUBBORN BASTARD

A high degree of stubborness is the chief charac-teristic of this type. He has certain fixed, dogmatic ideas about the right and wrong way of doing things; to try and change his mind at times seems like an impossible task. He is apt to pout and not communicate for long periods of time because he feels someone has treated him unjustly. He has a great deal of difficulty emphasizing or understanding other people's feelings and relating them appropriately. He is basically a loner who has tended to shut out the rest of the world. His stubborness, of course, carries over into his treatment, and he relates to the psychiatrist in much the same way. Less competent shrinks are apt to be fooled by this guy, thinking they are really communicating with him when he is merely paying lip service to what they are saying. The Stubborn Bastard makes no real changes in terms of his actual life. It is with this type of patient that a competent psychiatrist must become extremely active and firm in order to get the attention focused on the real problems. Sometimes it is not until such a patient becomes very angry with the therapist that he can begin to relate in a meaningful way. Therapy will be prolonged because his innate stubbornness resists all efforts at change. If you can hang in there long enough with this kind of guy, though, his resistance will eventually begin to break down. I must confess that, at any given time, I would prefer having only a couple of them in treatment. They sure can wear you down.

THE BULLSHIT ARTIST

This patient comes into the office presenting himself as a person who fully understands all of his problems and the reasons for them. He tries to snow the psychiatrist into agreeing with him. He tries to take over control of his own therapy and will even point out some of the problems of the psychiatrist. He always has to be one-up on the therapist and anticipate his every move. He fears even the slightest degree of passivity or dependence upon the doctor. The competent psychiatrist, of course, tends to take this in his stride and is not threatened by such manipulations. He will point out to the patient very simply and matter-of-factly what he is doing. He will gradually gain the patient's confidence so that the latter does not have to be so aggressively defensive. The Bull-shit Artist can then usually begin to relax and get involved in treatment in a positive way. For the first time in his life, he realizes that his line of crap not only doesn't work, but is the very thing that has been getting him into trouble for so many years in the past.

THE INTELLECTUALIZER

Another negative attitude or defense mechanism that tends to interfere with the smooth development of a positve working relationship is that which consists of using ideas and thoughts to cover up feelings. Usually above average in intelligence, this patient tries to impress the therapist with how smart he is. He relates to the therapist more as a student of psychology than as a patient. He constantly makes interpretations of his own behavior, which he thinks will outsmart the therapist, rather than get down to the business at hand. Some Intel-lectualizers are able to get closer to a feeling level when their behavior is pointed out to them. Others, however, play the intellectual games indefinitely. Any psychiatrist, of course, who gets caught up in such a game in an effort to prove his own brilliance ultimately loses the patient. The latter eventually realizes that nothing significant is being accomplished, and he will quit treatment. The com-petent psychiatrist must help such a person realize that he is not there to prove how brilliant he is, but that he comes to the doctor's office for help with his emotional problems. Forcefully discouraging such intellectual games is the first priority of the treatment. Obviously compensating in this misguided fashion for his sense of inferiority, the patient can be a hard nut to crack. If he combines this defense with that of the Stubborn Bastard or the Bullshit Artist, the therapist has on his hands the equivalent of two or three patients in one.

THE INJUSTICE SEEKER

This is the kind of person who always feels he is being exploited by some person or group. Whether it is a parent, spouse, boss, or organization, he will vigorously contend that others are taking advantage of him. At first glance, it may appear that he is corect. On a closer inspection, however, it generally turns out that he is unconsciously and repetitively setting things up this way. He structures his relationships in such a way that others will exploit him. This enables him to then go through life blaming others for his own shortcomings. He creates his own enemies in order to have a constant scapegoat for his feelings. If the psychiatrist is not careful, he, too, will be blamed by the Injustice Seeker. The search for a scape-goat is as old as man himself. This ancient tribal custom has many contemporary forms, including the radical ele-ments on both sides of the political scene.

THE MASTER OF INDECISION

This person feels that he has a major decision to make. Like an insect frozen by fear if he moves in any direction, he seems unable to move off dead center and make up his mind. He wants to be told what to do, but if the shrink tries, the Master of Indecision will resist him with all his might. He is stuck in the psychological posi-tion of baiting people into trying to give him advice just so he can refuse that advice. He chases his own tail in progressively smaller circles. He can think of endless reasons for both doing and not doing something, but he can't bring himself to do anything. He is perpetually on the horns of a dilemma. This degree of indecision is never easy to treat. Some people, unfortunately, live this way for years, unable to make any decision about what to do with themselves, either in terms of marriage or vocation. For fear of making a mistake, they can procrastinate forever. The responsibility involved is more than they are prepared to handle, and they can't trust themselves or anyone who tries to advise them. The first stage of therapy is quite prolonged in such cases.

These patient types may exist in relatively pure form or be combined in various proportions. It is not usual for an Intellectualizer to also be a Master of Indecision, or a Masochist to display characteristics of an Injustice Seeker. In any case, one can see why the psychiatrist's work is very tedious.

PSYCHIATRISTS ARE HUMAN

Many patients, after they have seen me a few times, will make some such comment as "Doctor Lazarus, I don't understand how you can possibly sit there all day long listening to one patient after the other tell you about their problems. I just don't see how you do it!" I must confess here that I usually answer this question rather glibly with a statement like, "That's why I went through medical school, internship, and three years of psychiatric residency training. You learn through all this and a few years of experience how to avoid letting other people's problems get under your skin. You learn how to forget your work when you go home at night and come back the next day refreshed. You learn how to be personally involved with each individual patient, but not to the point where it becomes a problem for you." This is not the complete truth. I don't care how competent the psychiatrist becomes over the years. As a matter of fact, if he becomes so confident that he is never perplexed or never questions his own work, he probably isn't half as competent as he thinks he is. The practice of psychiatry *is* a nerve-racking business to a certain extent. Ask any psychiatrist's wife; she'll tell you. After all, she is the one to whom he unloads the unfinished business of the day. There are times when, after a hectic day at the office, the first thing I do is stretch out on my couch and think out loud. Who else would listen except my wife?

The more I think about it, the more I believe that it is necessary for a psychiatrist who wants to be competent in his field to have a wife who can listen to him occasionally discuss some of the fine points of his involvment with patient's problems—a wife who can just listen and, at times, make some common-sense remarks that frequently help the guy put things in better perspective. Needless to say, I never identify any patients by name, and she never discusses the problems with anyone else. Psychiatrists are human. If shrinks were more open with each other in terms of discussing their cases, they wouldn't have to use their wives for this purpose. By all means, don't marry a psychiatrist if you do not want to hear about other people's problems!

It's not hard to understand why tensions can build up even in the most competent among us. Just imagine, if you will, a morning composed of sessions with one Hungry Mouth, one Stubborn Bastard, one Miracle Seeker, and one Bullshit Artist. These patient types are not so rare that such combinations don't occur with periodic regularity—and with not even one Seducer to liven things up a bit during the whole morning!

However, these stereotyped patients are perhaps the least of a good psychiatrist's problem. What really builds up is the constant grind of paying complete attention to every word, idea, and feeling that every patient utters during the course of an eight-hour workday, at least five days a week. It's not just paying close attention to all the things that people talk about, it's trying to figure out the proper strategy to meet the needs of each individual at all times. This is what takes its toll. At the same time, this is what provides the essential and unique fascination about the field of psychiatry. One has to constantly exercise all of the ingenuity he can possibly muster up from day to day. For the competent psychiatrist, at least, it is a tremendously challenging and creative field, but trying to be creative all the time is both nerve-racking and exhausting. Anyone who says different is either putting you on or kidding himself.

I remember a young lady I saw about a year ago. No matter what I said to her, no matter how considerate I tried to be, she'd find at least three or four reasons why I was completely wrong. This kind of relationship continued for several months before things began to change for the better. I remember making the remark to her once that she seemed awfully difficult to please and that there must be some good reasons for this. She immediately replied, "Of course there are good reasons for it. Do you think I'd be this way if there weren't? Do you have to be a psychiatrist to make such profound observations?" In many respects, I agree with one of my better teachers who made the comment once that the basic function of the psychiatrist is to serve as a professional scapegoat. If this is true, and I am sure there is considerable merit to the observation, it would certainly explain a lot of the harassment that any psychiatrist has to deal with.

Besides all that, there is the constant challenge of having to re-evaluate one's goals with any particular patient. Recently, a woman who had come to me for the treatment of depression, after beginning to feel better, asked whether or not she should continue treatment. She wanted to resolve certain other problems that were only very remotely related to the initial depression for which she sought help. I remember having to switch gears mentally, to put her in a different perspective so that I could see her now as a new and really different patient. It took me quite awhile to recognize my approach to this patient so that I could answer her questions intelligently. It's not unusual in treating patients that once you put out the initial fire, a new fire develops or some whole new set of emotional conflicts comes to the surface that needs further work. The psychiatrist frequently has to change his formulation of the patient's problems as the patient himself changes. There may be some psychiatrists who can do this automatically. I am not one of them.

I remember when the whole drug thing started with the kids, and they began coming for psychiatric help. My first exposure to a seventeen-year-old, bushy-haired, unshaven, barefoot, saintly appearing speed freak was traumatic as hell. I didn't know whether to shit or get off the pot, and it was difficult for me to conceal my bewilderment from him. Somehow I managed to pull myself together and get down to business, but things did not progress as smoothly with him then as they would today. After repeated exposure to such new forms of deviation from the norm, I can keep my cool and remain fairly objective most of the time.

The new sexual patterns that have emerged in recent years have also thrown us psychiatrists for a loss temporarily. Initially, like our peers in other fields, we tended to judge this behavior morally and ethically. Living together prior to marriage, for example, we tended to regard simply as poor impulse control as a result of immaturity and weak ego structure. We know now that to oversimplify things in this way is patently ridiculous. The psychiatrist, unlike most people, can't just take his time adapting to basic changes in social customs. He has to get with it very quickly if he is to be of significant help to his patients. He not only has to know what is acceptable behavior in our society, he has to know also what deviations from tradition are part of the changing social and cultural milieu. Society changes just as the individual does, and it's changing faster today than ever before.

Another problem that constantly makes the psychiatrist's work difficult is dealing the the potentially or actually suicidal patient. If you believe, as I do, that suicide is always preventable, you can understand why the responsibility of the psychiatrist will at times weigh rather heavily. It's not always feasible to lock up the suicidal patient. It's not always necessary to do so. On the other hand, it's not true, as some psychiatrists seem to think, that if you have a postive transference going with the patient, that this in itself will necessarily deter him from future suicide attempts. With these patients, it is doubly important that you say the right thing at the right time. Further, the old maxim stating that if someone really wants to bump himself off there is no way to stop him, is also nonsensical. He can be stopped, he should be stopped, and he must be stopped. That doesn't mean I'm going to go into a deep, dark depression if one of my patients does the dirty deed. It does mean though that I will spend some time trying to figure out why and how it happened and what I might have done to prevent it from happening.

There are other kinds of problems that come up. I remember seeing one couple for a marital problem where I couldn't help but identify with the wife against the husband. She was beautiful, as apparently normal as a person could be, but helpless to cope with a husband who was two-timing her and trying to conceal it. It took all of the forbearance I could muster to restrain from asking her why the hell she was married to a bum like that. I finally managed to resolve the problem by seeing them separately for a while. He finally came clean and discussed the situation openly, decided he was really in love with his wife, and gave up his extracurricular activities. To the best of my knowledge, they lived happily ever after, but, even then, I couldn't help but wonder why the hell she stayed with him.

It works in reverse also. I remember another couple where the wife was openly flouting her marital vows and seeking a divorce. She was terribly immature and emotionally incapable of motherhood. The husband was a handsome, conscientious, hard-working, virile male who could have had his pick of women, but we wanted her and he got her—after a few months of treatment. So, we psychiatrists are human too. The only difference though is that we evaluate the needs of our patients as objectively as possible and refrain from making any snap judgments that would contradict the basic desires of those who come to us help. Obviously there are a few other differences too.

One of the things that really slays me is the way I see sick parents constantly undermining the self-esteem of their young children. Despite our best efforts, the children of our patients sometimes have to pay the price for their parents' illnesses. If you think this is easy for a conscientious psychiatrist to live through, then you not only need psychiatric treatment yourself, you need an exchange blood transfusion from a real human being. There is a host of other problems equally difficult for a psychiatrist. The purpose of this book, however, is not for me to discuss the personal problems of my daily work so much as to inform you of how I think the public can get more for its money out of the field generally and help improve the standards of psychiatric practice.

CHAPTER **6**

Commonly Asked Questions

WHAT FOLLOWS IS a sampling of the questions I am most frequently asked. They represent the persistent misgivings that many people still rightfully have about the field of psychiatry. So many shrinks are apt to be evasive when these questions are asked or to dodge the basic issues involved, whereas the competent psychiatrist must literally open himself up full in an effort to completely dispel the person's anxiety and provide the kind of reassurance that is so vital to the progress of a therapeutic relationship. There simply is no room in psychiatry for wishy-washy, half-baked answers to valid questions. The answers must be very straight and direct. Any kind of pussyfooting around here on the part of the therapist warrants an attitude of suspicion and cautious mistrust.

Does a psychiatrist really ever cure anyone?

Not only do psychiatrists cure people but they frequently do so in a very dramatic way in fewer than ten sessions. When I say the person is cured, I mean he no longer has the symptoms that led him to seek help; he has resolved the underlying conflicts that led to the development of the symptoms in the first place, and in the process of treatment, has become a happier and more productive human being. Furthermore, when you do get a cure, it is extremely unlikely that that person is ever going to develop the same kind of illness in the future.

You know this because the patient has achieved a certain amount of insight, both intellectual and emotional. The conflicts have been digested to the point where the kind of situation that led to the patient's illness will now be handled in an entirely different way by the person. Instead of internalizing the difficulties and the frustrated emotions involved, the feelings will be expressed openly, honestly, and in a constructive fashion. The blocks to communication will have been removed. The person becomes more confident of himself and more optimistic about his ability to deal with the kinds of issues from which he had previously hidden. He has a heightened capacity to objectively evaulate human relationships and consequently can better assess his own role and responsibility. He will then be able to act in accordance with the realities of any situation rather than be dominated by his previous fears and fantasies.

Being cured does not mean that the individual will never get upset or angry, only that he will do so when it is clearly indicated. In short, the person will be more human and less stereotyped in his reactions. It is not true that the fully analyzed person is one who always maintains his cool and never gets his feathers ruffled. He will be cool and rational much of the time, but he will not hesitate to express his feelings on subjects that touch him deeply. So the answer is most affirmatively yes; some patients are cured, assuming, of course, that they receive competent psychiatric assistance.

I feel so miserable. I don't see how talking can help me. How can talking help anyone?

It's no wonder you feel so wretched. You never really learned how to talk to people. You never learned the most important lesson in human life: how to use words to express feelings. It is primarily through verbal communication that one frustrated, anxious, human being can impart these feelings to another, can let the other person in to share the misery. You turn all your feelings back upon yourself instead of letting them out, instead of sharing them with other people and thus understanding them yourself. You're depressed and miserable because you either never learned how or you've forgotten how to do this.

Let's take the most common example. When a child is growing up and feels frustrated or deprived, he cries; he lets the protecting parent know that something is wrong so that the parent can comfort, soothe, and fulfill the frustrated need of the moment. As the child develops beyond those early years and learns how to use language and his own powers of self-observation, he learns how to identify his own frustrations and problems and then bring them to the attention of the parent. Through the mechanism of a healthy parent-child relationship, the child learns how to express feelings in a way that will meet his basic needs. Your lack of confidence in talking as a vehicle for expressing emotions and fulfilling needs indicates certain unresolved problems in this area of your growth and development. If you really want to get well, you'll stop focusing primarily on how miserable you feel and begin to identify in words and feelings the real

problems that you are having in your everyday life. Now
let's get down to business: quit feeling so sorry for yourself that you don't even want to talk about your situation.

> *Aren't there some patients who are so chron-
> ically ill that they will never really be fully inde-
> pendent? People who will always have to be
> cared for by their families or will have to be on
> welfare the rest of their lives. These people can't
> be cured can they?*

That is true. There are a number of patients who
have been sick for many years who remain dependent on
their families or society at large. Some remain in hospitals and give the definite impression that no amount of
time or psychiatric attention would significantly alter the
degree of disability which they suffer. Others see psychiatrists intermittently in order to be maintained on medication, thus avoid the need for hospitalization.

Obviously we are talking here about the more severe
forms of mental illness. The regrettable fact of the matter
is that a large number of these people were not brought
to psychiatric attention soon enough in the course of their
illness to prevent this. For a number of them, illness
has become a way of life. These victims should not be
pitied nor should they be despised. They simply represent
failures in human adaptation. In actual fact, they are
symbolic not of their own personal failures but of society's failure to properly identify the problems at an early
enough stage in the development of the illness to provide
the kind of competent psychiatric help that I have been
describing. I certainly, however, would not pronounce
anyone incurable unless he has had a very thorough and
competent psychiatric evaluation. In my experience, I
have found that it is not at all unusual to see a patient
who looked relatively hopeless during the first interview,

begin to blossom forth rather surprisingly after a few sessions. And, on the contrary, I have seen many patients who appeared at first blush to have relatively minor problems but when seen over a period of time turned out to have rather deep-rooted and relatively inflexible disturbances.

How come you don't have a reclining couch in your office? I thought I came here to be psychoanalyzed.

Psychoanalysis as a form of treatment has been found to be too time consuming, too expensive, too impractical, and far too unproductive in terms of improvement or cure. Psychotherapy today consists of a face-to-face encounter between patient and therapist. The competent psychiatrist will deal only with those areas of a person's life which need to be discussed in any depth. For most people, there is a very pragmatic need to conserve time and money and still get the best results possible. The prone position and the daily sessions serve only to prolong the therapy, assure the analyst of his continued financial security, and endlessly complicate the entire process of treatment.

I have a terrible fear of crowds and I am also very fearful of being alone. Do you believe that there is a sexual explanation for all problems and specifically do you think my problem is basically a sexual one?

No, it simply is not true that all problems can be explained on a sexual basis. Though some of them can be, many cannot. It's perfectly conceivable to me that you may have a very adequate sexual relationship with your spouse and still have the problems you have mentioned. We are going to have to track down the origins of these two phobias without any preconceived notions about the causes. As a matter of fact, there are very few human problems that can be explained away on a strictly sexual basis. Most problems are multidetermined and have several causes, one of which may be sex. A lot of people have misinterpreted Sigmund Freud because he defines sex in a very loose fashion. But that would take us too far afield. Let's get down to the problem of your fears. When did you first begin having this kind of trouble?

What about the amount of time it takes? I read recently where the typical number of sessions in psychoanalysis ranged from 300 to 500 hours?

Competent psychotherapy takes anywhere from one hour to one hundred fifty hours. I see the vast majority of my patients only once a week. I am not referring now to hospital patients whom I see approximately three times a week. As far as outpatients are concerned, I see them sometimes two or three times a week as needed. With respect to the number of hours required, let me point out that there are three kinds of patients. With the first kind of patient, you average between ten and twenty hours of therapy. This is the person who has developed an acute problem or set of symptoms of recent origin and whose basic personality structure is relatively healthy. The second type of patient, who will require between thirty and fifty hours, has a long-term problem or set of symptoms and is basically trying to learn how to cope better with certain types of situations, both internal and external. He wants to understand the origins of his problems but is basically content to learn how to adjust better. The third type of patient requires in the neighborhood of 100-120 hours. Different goals are involved. He wants to effect a basic change within himself. His need is not to solve any single problem or illness of recent origin nor is it to learn how to cope more effectively with everyday life situations. Rather, he is attempting to bring about a complete change in the way he perceives himself and in the way he relates to other people. His problems may or may not be more deeply rooted than patients in the first two categories, but his goals are certainly more ambitious. For example, whereas previously he has always remained distant from other people and has entered into only shallow, artificial, human relationships, he now seeks to relate to people on a much deeper and intimate level. He wishes to alter his self-concept from a very mechanical or inadequate level to one of real warmth, depth, and versatility. Obviously such a job requires more time.

Are there some problems that may take only a few hours of treatment?

Yes, I see a number of people who fall into that category. For example, I recently saw a woman who, for the past several years, had felt that she had an ideal marriage. One day she happened to overhear the tail end of a conversation her husband was having with a woman. In the course of that conversation, he referred to this woman as "honey." The patient became panic-stricken at the thought that her husband could possible be having an affair with another woman. This thought stirred up many bitter memories of a past marriage in the course of which her ex-husband had frequently been unfaithful to her. She was so upset that she was unable to discuss the subject intelligently with her husband at the time. I saw this woman on two separate occasions, and we discussed in great detail the reasons for her overreacting in the way that she had. Within one week's time, she was able to understand her reaction, the relationship between her and her husband had returned to normal, and she has lived happily ever after.

Had this reaction gone untreated and had it been allowed to severely complicate the marital relationship, a number of psychiatric complications might have arisen. She might have become very depressed and possibly suicidal. The marriage might have ended in divorce. She might have developed a full-blown neurotic illness in relation to men generally. This kind of very abbreviated therapy happens with such regularity that one can only conclude that it is a myth that psychiatric treatment has to take a long time and has to be very expensive.

I am in a very stressful situation right now. I'm already 45 years old and now I have to pull up stakes and move my entire family. I am very nervous about it. It's beginning to affect my appetite and I'm not sleeping very well. Even though I have to make this move in less than a month, should I come in to see you? Will we have enough time to really accomplish anything?

A great deal can be accomplished in a month's time. If necessary, I will arrange to see you more frequently than just once a week, depending on how complex the problem really is. Since your reaction is directly related to this compulsory move, it will be quite easy to identify all of the factors responsible for your insecurity at this time. We will then be able to help you put the whole thing in much better perspective, rearrange your feelings in a more objective fashion, and help you decide how you want to deal with any of the problems that the move entails. Obviously, we are not going to deal at great length with your past history. We shall focus pretty much on the here-and-now situation in helping you come to terms with the move. This is what is generally known as "crisis intervention," and it has a very legitimate place in the field of psychotherapy. As a matter of fact, I would be very surprised if we couldn't wrap up the whole problem within the alloted time.

Is seeing a psychiatrist going to change me in some way? I don't really want to change that much. I just want to get over these uncomfortable feelings I have.

As a result of your treatment here, you will not change in any way that you do not want to change. When you are through with your treatment, you will still be the same basic person that you are right now. At any time during the treatment process, when we get into any of your hang-ups and you become fearful that I expect you to change in a way you do not desire, please let me know immediately and we will discuss it. Throughout your treatment, you should feel free to interrupt and ask me any questions or express any fears at any time. And I will try to allay your fears in every way possible. My job is not to force people to change, it is to help them deal with the problems for which they themselves want help. I certainly would not undertake to change the things you already like about yourself. So now, tell me what it is that you don't like.

I've been down in the dumps lately, but I think everyone gets depressed at times. How do you tell when you have exceeded the safety limit and really need to see a psychiatrist?

You have exceeded the safety limit when the feelings of depression don't seem to want to go away, when you feel unable to cope with the depression to the degree that it begins to interfere with your everyday life. Now, it is true that some people can't stand being depressed for even twenty-four hours. Others seem to have a greater tolerance and can remain somewhat depressed for days or even weeks at a time without feeling the need to yell for help. My main point is that as soon as the question arises in your mind regarding whether or not you need psychiatric help, it would be a good idea to get a check-up, because then, and only then, can you understand all of the factors involved in the development of your depressed state. What this will accomplish, at the very least, is to satisfy you that you do not have a serious problem. You may also learn how to deal with any future similar episodes. And you can utilize that session with the psychiatrist to discuss any aspect of your life about which you may be concerned.

A competent psychiatrist is not going to keep you coming back to him simply to add to his list of patients unless he feels it would be helpful for you to do so. Hopefully, you would be able to put this kind of visit to a psychiatrist in the same category as getting a routine medical checkup. Put very simply, not only is it true that a person does not have to be nuts to go see a shrink, he doesn't even have to be sick. Some objective feedback from a psychiatrist will help anyone to feel better about himself, to be more optimistic about the future, and to resolve any doubts he may have about his overall emotional state.

Due to a shortage of money I have been referred to group therapy. Is this a satisfactory substitute?

Group therapy is never a substitute for individual therapy. If your problem is primarily in the area of how

you relate to other people, you may well benefit considerably from group psychotherapy. Assuming that you
are not completely broke and heavily in debt, your problem should first be evaluated by a competent psychiatrist
who would then tailor-fit a treatment program to meet
your individual needs. I will frequently work out a combination of individual and group therapy in such a way as
to keep the expense to a minimum. In such cases, it may
not be necessary to see the psychiatrist every week or for
a full hour. A half-hour every other week may suffice in
your particular case. Group therapy, when properly conducted, can be very effective in the overall psychiatric
treatment. I do not feel though that group therapy should
ever be regarded as a complete substitute for individual,
psychiatric treatment.

*In my home town there are no psychiatrists but
there are one or two people who are psychologists or social workers. Would this be a satisfactory way of my getting help with my emotional
problems?*

First of all, you should check out the credentials of
these people. Make sure that they are graduates of accredited training programs. The psychologist should have
at least a master's degree from an accredited school and
preferably a Ph.D. Ph.D's are much less common among
social workers, and the master's degree is certainly sufficient. Second, whoever this person is, you should check
on whether he or she has a good working relationship
with one of the physicians in the community. Assuming
this to be the case, it is conceivable that the physician
could prescribe any needed medication while the
psychologist or social worker performed the actual psychotherapy. I realize that there are communities in which

one does not have a great deal of choice. Under such circumstances, you might be very pleasantly surprised to find that the person in question is quite competent indeed. If not, however, you might have to commute to a nearby city for the help you need.

Is there really such a thing as a completely normal person? Aren't we all a little freaky at times?

There are some people who conform to the norm and in that sense, they are normal people. Studies have indicated that as a group, they are rather boring, dull, uninspiring, and shallow in their way of life. Most of us do have certain neurotic tendencies that at times get the better of us. I think the important thing is not so much to be "normal," but rather to be as aware as possible of one's neurotic tendencies so that under circumstances of stress, one can prevent these tendencies from dominating the situation. Because of the nature of our society, this cannot always be done. Everyone has his breaking point. Furthermore, most people need to "blow off steam" periodically. They have a definite need at times to act silly and childish just for the fun of it. Finally, the type of person who goes around trying very hard to be normal and dignified all of the time is probably one of the most neurotic types of all.

I have the feeling that buried in my past somewhere are some very traumatic memories that I have repressed. Wouldn't hypnosis facilitate my conscious memory of these events and thus speed up my treatment?

In the course of your treatment, you will relearn how to express your feelings both in the present and in the

past. By focusing on hypnosis, you are trying to artificially bypass your problems, as if the doctor could in
some magical way extract them from you in the way a
surgeon would extract a diseased organ. Hypnosis has a
legitimate place in anethesia, in posthypnotic suggestion
for obesity, and other very specific conditions. In your
case, hypnosis would only be another form of mental
masturbation. Like so many patients who intellectualize
excessively, you are looking for some quick and easy
answer to solve your problems rather than dealing with
your real feelings. And before you ask me, the same goes
for "truth serum" or sodium amytal.

> *Do you ever come into physical contact with
> your patients, either to touch them in any way or
> possibly become even more intimate?*

I tend to follow a hands-off policy. I do occasionally
shake hands with a male patient when meeting him for
the first time. And I have no sympathy with any psychiatrist who literally prostitutes himself in the name of
trying to help his patients. He needs help with his own
problems and should not be let loose on the public as a
psychiatrist until he has received competent treatment
himself. The nature of the therapeutic relationship
through the expression of feelings provides all of the intimacy that any patient really requires. The competent
therapist never makes love to any of his patients, but he
does show his deep concern for their welfare.

> *I don't want to discuss that subject. It's too pain-
> ful. Why don't we just let the past be forgotten
> and go on to something else?*

While it is true that in some instances it is not necessary to dredge up painful memories from the past, in

your case I find that these particular memories are directly related to the reasons for which you sought help. Go right ahead and cry if you like. You'll probably find it quite helpful. I'm afraid you are simply going to have to trust my judgment in this respect. After all, that is one of the things you are paying me for.

Are these pills which you have prescribed habit forming?

The medication I have prescribed for you is neither habit forming nor addicting. I prescribed it for you because you need some relief from your symptoms in order to be better able to discuss and work through your real problems. Take the medication only as prescribed. If you do so and continue to work on your problems as you have been, your need for the medication will decrease over a period of time. If I feel that you are becoming overly dependent on it and using it merely as a crutch, I will let you know. This is very seldom the case with people like yourself who tend to take too little medication rather than too much.

My son was told by his counselor at school that because of his behavior he would have to be placed on Ritalin. Otherwise, they are going to suspend him. I don't know what to do.

You have done the proper thing. After you relate the history of the problem to me, I will check with the school and then see your son. I will then make a diagnosis and decide whether Ritalin should be included as part of his treatment. If the boy does in fact suffer from "the hyper-kinetic syndrome," we shall discuss the matter fully in terms of your relationship with him, his relationship to the people at school, his feelings about himself, and whether he needs any medication.

Isn't it risky for a child or even an adult to be on any of these medications since they may affect the body in some unknown way and the effects not show up for many years?

All of the medications that are generally prescribed have been tested thoroughly in the laboratory. Further, they have been in common use now for many years and though in some instances possible side effects do occur, they can be spotted early enough by the competent psychiatrist to prevent any kind of real damage. I personally have participated in several research projects in the area of psychopharmacology and am very keenly aware of the potential dangers involved. If I prescribed any given medication for you or your child, be sure to report to me any side effects that you think may be attributable to the drug. We will discuss it at the time, and I will then advise you as to the appropriate course of action. As you well know, a person can be allergic to any medication, whether it be aspirin, penicillin, or whatever. This should in no way deter you from taking any medication prescribed for you by a competent physician.

Do you regard electroshock therapy as an extraordinary form of treatment?

Yes, I do. Since the discovery of several antidepressant medications, the need for EST is practically nonexistent. In the past three years I have prescribed shock treatment in only two cases. In one case, the woman was terribly ill, was not responding to any of the medications I had prescribed for her, and was herself very deeply convinced that shock treatments were the only thing that would help her. She had had such treatments once before many years ago. I reluctantly acquiesced, but stopped after only three treatments because they were really not helping her. She, nevertheless felt that they did.

In the second instance, I prescribed shock therapy because nothing else seemed to be helping, and I'm happy to report that after six treatments, the patient did seem moderately improved. When you realize that this is only two out of the hundreds of patients I have seen during the past three years, it certainly makes one wonder if there really is a continuing indication for the use of electroshock therapy in any patients at all. In fairness to this form of treatment, let me say that with the use of pentothal anesthesia and Anectine as a muscle relaxant, the teatment need not be at all traumatic to the patient. He merely goes to sleep for a few minutes, wakes up somewhat disoriented, and then goes about his business within a half-hour. If the total number of treatments is restricted to under fifteen, we see very little, if any, persistent memory loss. However, as I say, the indications for its use today are practically nill.

You told me that the medication which you have prescribed has just recently come out on the market. I don't want to be a guinea pig. Do you as a psychiatrist prescribe a new medication on the basis of what the drug company itself says about it?

First of all, I am prescribing this new medication because none of the old standbys happen to work with you. Second, I have read the reports of independent investigators who have thoroughly evaluated the

medication in clinical trials. I generally do not trust what
the drug companies themselves say about the new medications in their advertisements.

*I read an article recently telling about the dan-
gers of a certain medication. The list of possible
harmful effects far exceeded the positive ones.*

Most medications have a long list of possible harmful
side effects. However, if it is prescribed by a competent
psychiatrist who understands the specific nature of your
problems, you can rest assured that he would not be
prescribing that medication for you unless he felt it was
definitely in your best interest. I ask my patients to call
me at the first sign of dicculty so that adjustments can be
made before any harm has really been done to the patient.
Considering the fact that the majority of psychiatric
patients do at one time or another take some form of medication, the relative percentage of cases in which one has
to stop the medication is extremely small. At the risk of
seeming to be terribly repetitious, I will again emphasize
the need to seek help from a competent psychiatrist.

*I know that my twelve-year-old son Johnny has
been experimenting with drugs. I am not sure
whether it has gone beyond the marijuana stage.
Can you help me deal with the problem?*

Yes, but first you have to make an appointment for
yourself. In the course of that interview with you, I will
get Johnny's history as well as the history of your relationship with him. It may well be that during our conversation, I will be able to advise you regarding the specific techniques you might use to promote better communication between Johnny and yourself. We will then

also explore the possibility of my need to see John. But, by no means should you drag Johnny in here with you at the time of our first appointment. That would be the quickest way to turn him off completely. If we decide that it would be desirable for me to talk with him, I will discuss with you how you should approach him on the matter.

> *My boy friend is the old-fashioned type. He thinks that after we are married I should do nothing but stay home, do the housekeeping, take care of the children, and be his personal slave. I want to pursue a career.*

I will want to talk to both of you as soon as possible. It is very important that before marriage you and he have a complete understanding on these matters. I have seen too many marriages break up simply because of this kind of disagreement. During our discussion, I will be able to determine how solid the relationship is between the two of you and what you can reasonably expect in the matter of being able to pursue a career. Your future happiness is at stake. Some men are too inflexible.

> *I suspect that my son is living with a girl in his apartment. I don't understand how he could possibly do such a thing to me. I have been terribly depressed ever since I called him late one night and she answered the phone.*

During your first appointment, I will determine the extent of your depression and then begin treatment. I will examine your relationship with your son in some detail. We can also discuss why you have reacted so violently when you don't even know for sure whether they are, in fact, living together.

I like to come home and have a few drinks after
work in order to relax. My wife just can't stand it
when I drink, and she raises hell with me. I've
reached the end of my rope. We have been mar-
ried for thirty years and if she doesn't get off my
back soon, I am going to see my lawyer about
getting a divorce.

First I will want to see you to get the full history of
the marriage. I can then tell you how to approach your
wife so that she will come in and discuss her side of the
story. There are many possible explanations for her
behavior, and I would certainly hold off on seeing a lawyer until we have had an opportunity to review both sides
of the situation fully. Usually such problems can be
easily resolved when the real problems are identified
and treated.

For the past six months I have been so tired I
can't even do my housework. Furthermore, I
become very irritable over minor things. My
doctor checked me physically but couldn't find
anything wrong. I do have a chronic urinary
tract infection which he is treating with anti-
biotics, but I feel he is overlooking something.
I really don't see any sense in coming to see you.

Set up an appointment after I have had a chance to
review your case history with your doctor. I can assure
you that I will keep an open mind and not assume that all
of your problems are psychological. I will review your
case history with you in some detail, from both the physical and the emotional points of view. I will then advise
whether further medical evaluation is indicated. It may
surprise you to know that a competent psychiatrist is

frequently instrumental in making a physical diagnosis as well as a psychiatric one.

> *I have all kinds of physical complaints. I have headaches and stomachaches. Sometimes I can't catch my breath. I have both constipation and diarrhea and sometimes I get so dizzy I can hardly stand up. I have been to six different specialists in the past three months, and three of them told me I needed a psychiatrist.*

It is true that psychological problems can and do affect the body in many ways. It is quite possible that all of your physical symptoms are due to chronic nervous tension that finds its outlet through the autonomic nervous system. Only after I have seen you and had a chance to explore your life in detail will I be able to give you a final opinion. Since you have seen so many other specialists in the field of medicine, it is about time you saw a psychiatrist.

> *I seem to be doomed to failure when it comes to men. I go out with them for a while and then inevitably they all find some reason to quit me. I'm so horny now I could scream. Can you help me?*

Your problem of inability to maintain a lasting relationship with a member of the opposite sex certainly needs to be explored. There are many possible reasons for this kind of difficulty. However, don't expect the psychiatrist to satisfy your immediate sexual needs himself no matter how horny you may feel.

My husband just doesn't know how to make love to me. We've been married for five years, and all

*he wants to do is to hop on and off, satisfying his
own sex drive and treating me as if I were nothing but a hole. It's no wonder I'm getting frigid
toward him.*

Set an appointment with my secretary at your earl-
iest convenience so that I can get the whole history of
your sexual difficulties. I will then be able to determine in
what ways you may be contributing to the problem.
Don't make the mistake of trying to discuss the problem
with your husband while you are having relations. Remember that a stiff dick can't carry on a lengthy conversation. After seeing you, I will arrange to see your husband in order to find out what his problems are. I will
then see both of you and, assuming that you are both
willing to cooperate, we can get to the bottom of the
problem and figure out how it can best be resolved.

*For many years I have had a fear of being alone,
but it seems to be getting worse. I am imposing
on my husband and friends to the point where I
can't stand to be alone at all. Is it too late for me
to change now after all this time?*

The fact that you have allowed this phobia to go on
for such a long time certainly makes it more difficult to
treat. Although I can't guarantee you any positive results,
I would urge you to come in and see me as soon as possible. If you are now really determined to get over this
fear, I may be able to help you. One part of your therapy
will be to purposely stay alone for increasingly long periods of time beginning with only a few minutes. In other
words, as we gradually learn the reasons for your phobia and begin dealing with them, you are going to have
to begin practicing being alone under my direction.

I have been a homosexual for the past several years, but I have also occasionally enjoyed a heterosexual relationship. I don't think I can go on this way much longer. Can you help me?

The fact that you are bisexual means that you have the capacity to enjoy sexual relationships with the opposite sex. This is a big step forward in your attempt to overcome the problem of homosexuality. The success of your treatment will depend on several factors including the strength of your motivation to change and the reasons for the development of your homosexuality.

I have a terrible temper. My wife and I will have an argument, and I'll really blow my stack. Then I feel terribly ashamed of myself. She is now threatening to leave me. Can you help me learn how to control my temper?

It is important for you to realize two things at the outset. First, your problem is going to take several months to resolve. Second, I will insist that you keep your appointments regularly and not drop out of treatment simply because you happen to feel better for the moment. In other words, if your wife removes the threat because your behavior improves temporarily, I don't want you to believe, on that basis, that you are cured. This kind of problem does not go away overnight no matter how competent the psychiatrist might be. If you yourself really want to change and will do the work expected of you in your treatment then I may be able to help you. Assuming your request is not merely an attempt to bribe your wife into staying with you, we'll get along fine.

I have a cousin who lives in Philadelphia. He has already seen three psychiatrists but without

*any significant improvement. Would it be possible
for you to treat him?*

I dare say there are more than a few competent psychiatrists in a city the size of Philadelphia. If your cousin
will follow carefully the precepts laid down in this book.
I think he can get adequate treatment where he is.

I am currently treating a patient who lives two thousand miles away. He was very dissatisfied with his previous
psychiatric treatment and, quite by chance, happened to
read an article I had written on his kind of illness. In a very
determined way, he managed to contact me by phone,
despite the fact that I had moved twice since writing the
article. I have been treating him by means of cassette tapes.
He records a tape, sends it to me, and then I record my
responses.

If anyone had told me a year ago that you could
actually treat someone in this way, I would have been
cynical at best. Strange as it may seem, the guy is showing
definite signs of improvement. One of the reasons for the
treatment being effective in his case is that he appears
to be more comfortable talking to a tape recorder than he
is to the doctor directly. Somehow, it is less threatening
that way. He doesn't have to compete with me as he probably did with the face-to-face psychiatrist. Also, there was
a built in positive relationship because he was so impressed
by the article. He felt it demonstrated more understanding
of him than anyone else had ever shown. A very unique
situation surely, but one that possibly has some general
application. It is probably not true that face-to-face contact between patient and therapist is always essential. The
odd part of it is that I feel that I know him at least as well
as I know any of the patients whom I see regularly in the
office. Needless to say, there are also some disadvantages
involved in this form of treatment.

*As you can see Doctor, my wife is extremely
disturbed. I think she should be hospitalized as
quickly as possible, don't you?*

Yes sir, I do. I would like her to be hospitalized on the
supportive care unit of St. Joseph's Hospital. As you know,
St. Joseph's is not a psychiatric hospital, and the supportive care unit handles general medical and surgical
patients as well as psychiatric patients. We will thus avoid
the stigma of placing her in a psychiatric hospital since
her illness does not really require that. After she is admitted, I will examine her in greater detail and prescribe
a treatment routine which will include medication, psychotherapy, specifically tailored therapy by the nurses and
attendants, as well as occupational and recreational programs. You will be interviewed by the Family Counseling
Service at the hospital and if you have any questions about
any aspects of the treatment, feel free to call on me.
According to my secretary, your insurance will cover most
of the cost of hospitalization. You can anticipate that your
wife will be in the hospital approximately three weeks. If
you wish to speak with me further, I will be at the hospital
at about 5:00 P.M. to examine your wife and write orders
on her.

Can you really prevent mental illness?

Yes, by detecting problems at a very early stage of
development, you can frequently avoid serious difficulties
later. But in addition to early detection, I am in favor of
large-scale screening programs. Premarital screening, for
example, would help avoid some of the disastrous marriages that are entered into so freely.

I recently had occasion to treat a woman who become
psychotic shortly after the birth of her first child. She had

never previously been exposed to young infants. Her illness first manifested itself in relation to a tremendous fear of bathing the newborn baby lest she hurt it in some way. Had she participated in one of the programs on the care and feeding of new born infants during her pregnancy, I think there is a very good chance that she might have avoided her entire illness. Though this may sound like an oversimplification to you, I can assure you that it is not. In all other respects this person was basically a very healthy individual.

Another big problem area is that of retirement. So many people retire today who are completely unprepared psychologically. I sincerely believe that people can be prepared so that some of the disastrous consequences of retirement can be avoided.

A woman recently consulted me because she felt she was a few pounds overweight. You'd certainly never have known it from looking at her, but we used the hour to review her life in great detail looking for areas of conflict that might have led to serious difficulty. It was a psychiatric checkup. We discussed a minor problem she was having with her family at the time, and then I was able to reassure her that she had no serious hang-ups that required psychiatric treatment. For this she was most grateful.

The whole area of preventive psychiatry has not yet been significantly explored. Ideally, I would be spending all of my time doing routine checkups and preventive work. Other shrinks would prefer to treat the really sick ones, but as I see it, the basic function of psychiatry is to put ourselves out of business. I would like to see the day when psychiatry becomes true mental hygiene rather than what it is now—mainly, last-ditch efforts to rescue people from their own private hell. Some of us now feel that we know enough to be able to do this, and we should have the chance.

*I don't think I can really afford private treatment
at all, other than a quick evaluation by you. Can
you then refer me to a public clinic for followup
treatment?*

I would like to discuss your exact financial situation
with you first to determine your ability to make a minimal monthly payment toward your therapy. I might be
able to handle your case by seeing you for only a half-hour
every other week. I may want to refer you either to a
social worker or a psychologist in private practice.
Strange as it may seem, most people who have an income
above the poverty level can afford psychiatric treatment.
More insurance policies today provide at least partial
coverage, in fact, many people have coverage without
realizing it. Also, your problem may be of such a nature
that you will require only a few sessions to get on the right
track. With the help of an occasional phone call after that,
and perhaps a letter to the family doctor, the job can frequently be completed at a very nominal cost. If we determine that you definitely cannot afford private treatment,
I will then refer you to one of the local community clinics.
Many patients seen at these clinics do luck out and get
fairly good therapy. The trouble, though, is that it depends
on luck.

In a public clinic, you are at the mercy of the organization, and it's definitely harder to establish the personal
kind of relationship that I, as a psychiatrist, rely so
heavily upon to produce good results. Any public organization, by virtue of its size, promotes a certain amount of
depersonalization that tends to undermine the development of this vitally important therapeutic relationship.
Another major problem of the public clinic that tends to
create all kinds of additional problems is that it is usually
run by the kind of psychiatrist who conceives of patients

as statistics rather than as separate human beings. These birds never quite get down to the nitty-gritty of patient problems and how they can best be dealt with on a clinical level. That doesn't mean that some members of the staff may not be excellent therapists and take the kind of personal pride in their work that is so necessary in this business. Let me point out that twelve of my fifteen years in the field of psychiatry have been spent in public institutions on a full-time basis, so I know whereof I speak. If we have to go the route of a public clinic, I will personally try to expedite your seeing the right person.

Regarding the relationship of psychiatry and religion, what if any conflict is there between them, and how can it be resolved?

Psychiatry has a quarrel with only those forms of religion which emphasize the doctrine of original sin. Any belief that tends to focus on the idea that man is inherently evil conflicts with the basically humanistic approach to problems that psychiatrists must follow. After all, patients come to us mainly because they feel they are evil, and this in turn leads them to feel anxious and depressed. If any religion tends to reinforce a patient's pathological belief that he is essentially no good, then I, as a psychiatrist, must try to disengage the patient from that kind of belief, no matter what its original source.

Do you believe in women's lib?

While I believe that women have the right to equal employment opportunities and equal pay for the same job done by men, and that women should not be regarded simply as sexual objects, I also believe that we are witnessing the development of an overreaction to male chauvinism. Both sexes need each other equally, and we must learn to treat each other with mutual respect. It is still very important for women to remain feminine— feminine in the sense of being in close touch with their feelings, being able to express those feelings in soft and gentle ways and at the same time, consciously trying to please their boy friends or their husbands in a way that only women can. She in turn has the right to expect the male of the species to knock himself out to please her. The Victorian stereotype is out, but it is being replaced by a much more mature concept of male-female relationships. When you are working out the problem of your own feminine identity here in treatment, please feel free to interrupt me whenever you think I'm being chauvinistic in any way so that we can discuss it from all points of view.

To whom do you go when you need help? Or are you so perfect that you don't need that sort of thing?

Like everyone else, I need to discuss my problems with someone from time to time and I do so regularly. When the problem involves my work with a patient, I usually seek out a competent colleague and discuss the problem with him in an informal way.

My mother is getting terribly senile. It's becoming increasingly difficult for me to live with her. Is it sometimes necessary to have your own mother committed to a mental hospital?

Commitment is always a last resort and is seldom necessary. In the past five years, I have participated in only two commitments. One was a case of a seventy-five-year-old gentleman who, being extremely irrational, felt

compelled to kill himself, and made several serious efforts
to do so. He was completely unmanageable at home and
simply could not be talked into voluntary admission. It
was a lifesaving measure and, with competent treatment,
he was cured within six weeks. The second instance was
that of a forty-five-year-old housewife who had become
addicted to practically any barbiturate or narcotic that
she could lay her hands on. In addition, she had illegally
forged one or more prescriptions. She could not be con-
tained in an open hospital since she was constantly smug-
gling drugs into the place and, on one occasion, came very
close to death by overdose. I saw to it that she was committed, again as a last resort, and simply because she was
so very intractable. I feel that the commitment process
should be avoided whenever possible, and in my experience it can be in ninety percent of cases. To deprive someone of his fundamental human rights even when he is
ill is not a responsibility ever to be taken lightly. Now, tell
me about your mother and what kind of treatment she has
been receiving for her condition.

*Is it true you told my daughter when she was
here last time that she didn't have to do anything
I said? Since she has been coming to see you,
she seems to have lost all respect for me and
doesn't seem to care how much she hurts my
feelings.*

The primary goal of my work with your daughter has
been to try to help her become an individual who can
stand on her own two feet. All of her life she has felt
smothered and overprotected by you. Whenever she has
had feelings that were somewhat different from your own,
she felt constrained to keep those feelings buried and not
to let you know how she really felt. It should not be

surprising to you that as her treatment progresses she will at times express some very angry feelings, even when they may not be indicated. This is a necessary transitional phase for her to go through in order to become the mature person that I am sure you wish her to be. When she reaches that point, you will be able to respect her more as an adult and she will respect you more. Only then will the past be forgotten and forgiven and hopefully, the two of you will form a new relationship that will be built on a much more solid foundation. Please call me again if any questions should arise about my treatment of your daughter and, if necessary, set an appointment for yourself so we can discuss the problems from your own point of view in more detailed fashion. That might be helpful for both you and your daughter.

EPILOGUE

THOUGH I REALIZE I have not answered all of the questions about psychiatry, I hope that you, the reader, have achieved a little better understanding of what is involved in the difference between competent and incompetent treatment. Though I have oversimplified certain issues, I hope I have shed some light on them, e.g., who needs a psychiatrist, how to select one, and how to tell if the therapy is progressing as it should. That treatment does not have to be prolonged, that it does not have to be very expensive, and that most human problems are soluable are further propositions to which this book is dedicated. Furthermore, psychiatric illness can be prevented, and if only one person seeks help before his problem reaches pathological proportions, as a result of reading this book, I will feel justified in its writing.

Herbert R. Lazarus, M.D.